COVID-19 Vaccines - Current State and Perspectives

Edited by Ibrokhim Y. Abdurakhmonov

Published in London, United Kingdom

COVID-19 Vaccines - Current State and Perspectives
http://dx.doi.org/10.5772/intechopen.101006
Edited by Ibrokhim Y. Abdurakhmonov

Contributors
Madhurima Roy, Charuta Shrotriya, Irina Magdalena Dumitru, Wilson Lewis Mandala, Mohamed Khalis, Oumnia Bouaddi, Chakib Nejjari, Harshal Ashok Pawar, Aditya Manivannan Iyer, Kasturi Mahesh Tawde, Jaeyoung Kim, Nikita Thapa, Shahlo Turdikulova, Dilbar Dalimova, Alisher Abdullaev, Muzaffar Muminov, Erkin Musabaev, Bakhodir Yusupaliev, Botir Kurbanov, Ibrokhim Y. Abdurakhmonov, Wang Ruyue, Amanda Izeli Portilho, Elizabeth De Gaspari, Mohan Kumar, V.L. Surya, Fangwu Chen, Gao Ya

First published in London, United Kingdom, 2023 by IntechOpen
IntechOpen is the global imprint of INTECHOPEN LIMITED, registered in England and Wales, registration number: 11086078, 5 Princes Gate Court, London, SW7 2QJ, United Kingdom

British Library Cataloguing-in-Publication Data
A catalogue record for this book is available from the British Library

Additional hard and PDF copies can be obtained from orders@intechopen.com

COVID-19 Vaccines - Current State and Perspectives
Edited by Ibrokhim Y. Abdurakhmonov
p. cm.
Print ISBN 978-1-80355-357-3
Online ISBN 978-1-80355-358-0
eBook (PDF) ISBN 978-1-80355-359-7

Meet the editor

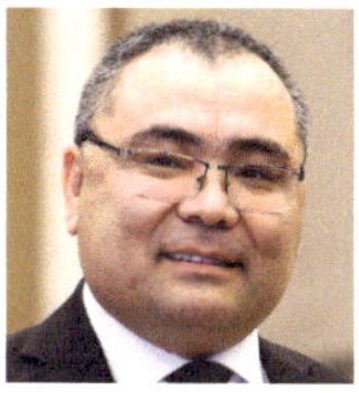

Ibrokhim Y. Abdurakhmonov received his BS in Biotechnology from the National University, Uzbekistan in 1997, an MS in Plant Breeding from Texas A&M University in 2001, and a Ph.D. in Molecular Genetics and DSc from the Academy of Sciences of Uzbekistan in 2002 and 2009, respectively. He founded the Center of Genomics and Bioinformatics of Uzbekistan in 2012. He received the 2010 TWAS prize and ICAC Cotton Researcher of the Year 2013 for his outstanding contribution to cotton genomics and biotechnology. Dr. Abdurakhmonov was elected as a fellow of The World Academy of Sciences (TWAS) in 2014 and a member of the Academy of Sciences of Uzbekistan in 2017. He was appointed Minister of Innovative Development of Uzbekistan in 2017. He was honored as the 2022 Ambassador of Silk Road Friendship (Individual) by the China International Culture Exchange Center (CICEC) and Global People Magazine for his contribution and leadership in fighting against the COVID-19 pandemic.

Contents

Preface

The severe acute respiratory syndrome coronavirus-2 (SARS-CoV-2) infection, which causes coronavirus disease 2019 (COVID-19), became the most devastating viral attack on humans of the past century. It caused unprecedented challenges for humanity, devastating the world economy, damaging human health, and taking many lives.

A COVID-19 vaccine is an antigenic molecule from the virus that helps the human body to generate an acquired immunity against the deadly SARS-CoV-2. At the beginning of 2020, there were no means to fight against this deadly virus. Thanks to previous studies on the structure and function of related viral genotypes causing severe acute respiratory syndrome (SARS) and Middle East respiratory syndrome (MERS), it was possible for the international research community to rapidly start investigations to develop COVID-19 vaccines, which were seen as the only way to minimize the harmful effect of this virus and reduce the death rate of infected people. Globally, leading pharmaceutical companies and centers of scientific research excellence as well as leading governments concentrated their attention and announced a major commitment to developing COVID-19 vaccines.

As a result of these efforts, in mid-to-late 2020, the first COVID-19 vaccine candidates were developed using traditionally attenuated/inactivated virus, recombinant adenovirus, and novel mRNA-based platforms. Vaccines were rapidly assessed, clinically trialed, and conditionally approved for emergency mass vaccination use. The vitality of these efforts reduced the spread of COVID-19 and minimized the severity of the illness and the number of deaths caused by SARS-CoV-2. Thanks to COVID-19 vaccines, humanity was able to prevent more than 20 million deaths per year, including those of 3 million children. As of October 2022, 11 vaccine types have been authorized by the World Health Organization (WHO) for emergency use. As a result, a total of about 13 billion doses of vaccine have been administered worldwide and more than 68% of the world population has received at least one dose of a COVID-19 vaccine. Although common side effects observed from the administration of COVID-19 vaccines such as soreness, redness, rash, inflammation at the injection site, fatigue, headache, and muscle/joint pains generally passed within a few days without medical treatment, some rare allergic reactions caused high public concern and vaccine hesitancy. Despite these reactions, even the severe ones, the benefit from COVID-19 vaccines remains higher than the observed risks.

At the same time, many open questions remain to be addressed. *COVID-19 Vaccines - Current State and Perspectives* has therefore brought together scientific contributions from the international research community covering the current status and latest advances in the development and application of the COVID-19 vaccine worldwide, as well as public perceptions, and the challenges associated with the post-immunization period. Chapters present a wide range of novel discussions on the current status of COVID-19 vaccine development, including: innovative outer membrane vesicles for novel vaccines; fast-tracked vaccine production and approval; side effects of COVID-19 vaccines with real-world examples on optic neuritis; future solutions involving the long-term COVID-vaccination program repurposing existing BCG and MMR vaccines; and public perception and vaccine hesitancy with clinical trial experience from some countries including Morocco and Uzbekistan. The country cases exemplify the challenges of each country's vaccine acquisition and application, which demanded a specific effort from their respective governments.

These peer-reviewed chapters will be an excellent addition to the almost 10,000 articles published to date on COVID-19 vaccines. I am confident not only that these discussions will be helpful to students and researchers in life sciences generally, and to healthcare specialists and medical doctors in particular, but also that they will help to determine current and future trends in the development of an effective vaccine against this novel coronavirus that is ruining the economy, human health, and lives. I wish to thank all the chapter authors for their efforts and invaluable contributions to this volume. I am grateful to the IntechOpen book department and Author Service Manager Ms. Sara Debeuc for the opportunity to work on this book project and for help with my editorial duties.

Ibrokhim Y. Abdurakhmonov
Center of Genomics and Bioinformatics,
Academy of Sciences of Uzbekistan,
Tashkent, Uzbekistan

Dedication

This edited volume is dedicated to all who contributed to the COVID-19 vaccine development, and to the COVID-19 frontline workers and fighters who worked long hours to reduce deaths during the pandemic.

Section 1

Introduction

Chapter 1

Introductory Chapter: Global Research Efforts toward the Development of COVID-19 Vaccines

Ibrokhim Y. Abdurakhmonov

1. Introduction

The sudden global spread of a novel coronavirus strain, infecting humans late in 2019, has created a deadly coronavirus disease 2019 (COVID-19), which has become a global threat to humanity [1, 2]. It started a new era of the COVID-19 pandemic with unprecedented socioeconomic challenges and societal crises due to long-term and periodic multiple lockdowns globally. The situation has been even more dangerous in the background of limited knowledge in understanding of the virus, its infection, and variability capacity as well as the lack of drugs and protocols of treatment. One of the most effective solutions against the COVID-19 virus in the pandemic has been a hope for rapid development of COVID-19 vaccines to overcome the global spread of virus infection via forming herd immunity. Thanks to the scientific efforts of world research communities, within a short time and with a fast-track project approach, several novel COVID-19 vaccines have been developed and made available for massive vaccination worldwide.

However, humanity still is in midst of this pandemic, and there is a need for better knowledge, understanding, technology, and innovative solutions to battle against this virus and its novel variants [e.g. see 1]. There were many challenges to rapidly developing COVID-19 vaccines against SARS-CoV-2, including designing immunogenic but nonallergic antigen molecules within a short time, proving experimentally in the appropriate *in vitro/in vivo* models, developing suitable protocols of vaccine administration, assessing the immune-response properties of candidate vaccine(s), conducting controlled and/or randomized the first to third phase safety and efficacy clinical trials involving regional and multicentral designs [1, 2].

Despite these challenges, scientific efforts have resulted in the development of several types of COVID-19 vaccines such as live-attenuated, mRNA-based, DNA-based, inactivated virus-based, and viral-vector-based vaccines. Some of the candidate vaccines have passed a rapid experimental validation in model animals with subsequent clinical studies for safety and suitability, leading to fast-track emergency use approvals (EUA) in many countries granted by World Health Organization (WHO). In particular, as of October 14, 2022, 11 candidate vaccines have been granted for emergency

#	Vaccine name	Company developed	No. trials/ countries	No. countries approved
1.	COVOVAX (Novavax formulation)	Serum Institute of India	7/3	6
2.	Nuvaxovid	Novavax	22/14	40
3.	Spikevax	Moderna	70/24	88
4.	Comirnaty	Pfizer/BioNTech	97/31	149
5.	Convidecia	CanSino	14/6	10
6.	Jcovden	Janssen (Johnson & Johnson)	26/25	113
7.	Vaxzevria	Oxford/AstraZeneca	71/33	149
8.	Covishield (Oxford/ AstraZeneca formulation)	Serum Institute of India	6/1	49
9.	Covaxin	Bharat Biotech	16/2	14
10.	Covilo	Sinopharm (Beijing)	38/17	93
11.	CoronaVac	Sinovac	40/10	56

Approval Source: extranet.who.int [3].

Table 1.
WHO-granted COVID-19 vaccines.

use by WHO [3]. Huge efforts were made toward assessment and making available of these vaccines for the massive population vaccination process, where one can see that 6–97 clinical trials in 1–33 countries have been conducted, leading to approval of emergency use of the particular vaccine(s) in 6–149 countries worldwide (**Table 1**).

The emergency use approvals of these WHO-granted vaccine candidates in each country have been specific, and vaccines have been administered in various combinations per availability and public perception. For instance, in Uzbekistan, we have had a specific experience with the COVID-19 vaccine development, clinical trial(s), acquiring/production, and massive vaccination process [4].

In Uzbekistan, we put concentrated efforts into the genetic characterization of SARS-CoV-2 genotypes in different periods of infection waves [5, 6] and have developed Uzbekistan's own PCR-based diagnostics tools, co-developed and jointly conducted third phase clinical trial for the new recombinant protein vaccine under China-Uzbekistan partnership program [4, 7]. We succeeded in co-localizing the production of recombinant vaccine jabs in the country. Further, we developed two new national vaccines based on pure recombinant protein injection and tomato-based edible COVID-19 vaccines, which are in the preclinical/clinical testing stages. Additionally, we studied and experimentally validated the new approach of obtaining immune cow and goat milk against SARS-CoV-2 [7].

Because of specific efforts from the Uzbekistan government, as of September 26, 2022, 71.9 million doses of seven types of COVID-19 vaccines have been used in the country. These are ZF-UZ-VAC2001 (as known Zifivax; China-Uzbekistan, pending WHO approval) – 48.2 million doses, Moderna (USA) – 10.7 million doses, Pfizer-BioNTech (USA) – 6.8 million doses, AstraZeneca (Great Britain) – 2.6 million doses, Sinovac (China) – 2.0 million doses, Sputnik V (Russia) – 1.3 million doses, and Sputnik light (Russia) – 345,000 doses.

According to the recommendation of the World Health Organization, the population over the age of 18 has mainly been vaccinated. The population of this age group in Uzbekistan was 21.5 million people, of which 98.5% are fully vaccinated and 76.6% (16.4 million people) received a booster dose. The distribution of administered vaccines was as follows: ZF-UZ-VAC2001 – 66.6%, Moderna – 15.5%, Pfizer-BioNTec – 8.9%, AstraZeneca – 3.8%, Sinovac – 2.7%, Sputnik V – 2.0%, and Sputnik light – 0.5%.

Today, "*68.3% of the world population has received at least one dose of a COVID-19 vaccine. A total of 12.83 billion doses have been administered globally, and 3.58 million are now administered each day. 23.3% of people in low-income countries have received at least one dose*" [8]. All these demonstrated the power and feasibility of scientific efforts and multinational collaborations in the timely development of effective vaccines against this most deadly infection of the past 100 years if concentrated attention is given and needed resources are provided [2]. There were common, fast-passing side effects with rare risky allergic reactions from the COVID-19 vaccination, but the benefits of COVID-19 vaccine administrations outweigh those risks.

However, there are more challenges ahead to address, including but not limited to the need for rapid development of novel vaccine types against emerging variants of concerns (VOCs), and the development of safe vaccination protocols for children and people with accompanying diseases. There is a need for addressing post-vaccination health issues, vaccine inequity, vaccine hesitancy, and vaccination ethics [9, 10] as well as for the establishment of large-scale production of high-quality and stable vaccines to make available needed jab volumes for all countries.

2. COVID-19 vaccine research focus during the pandemic

The scientific research articles devoted to the development and application of COVID-19 vaccines, retrieved from the *PubMed* database [11] using the keyword search of "*COVID-19 vaccine*," revealed a total of 9468 scientific publications as of October 2022 (**Figure 1**). Using Pubmed graphics and filtration tools, we observed that scientific results started to be published in 2020 (415 publications) and the

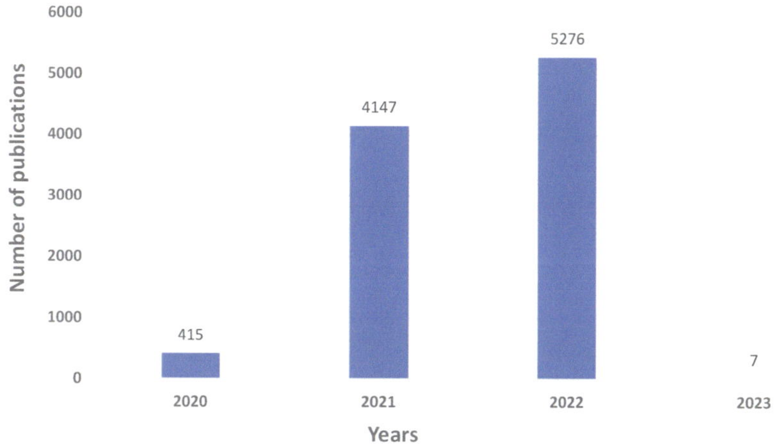

Figure 1.
PubMed [6] indexed scientific publications, retrieved using the "COVID-19 vaccine" keyword on October 12, 2022.

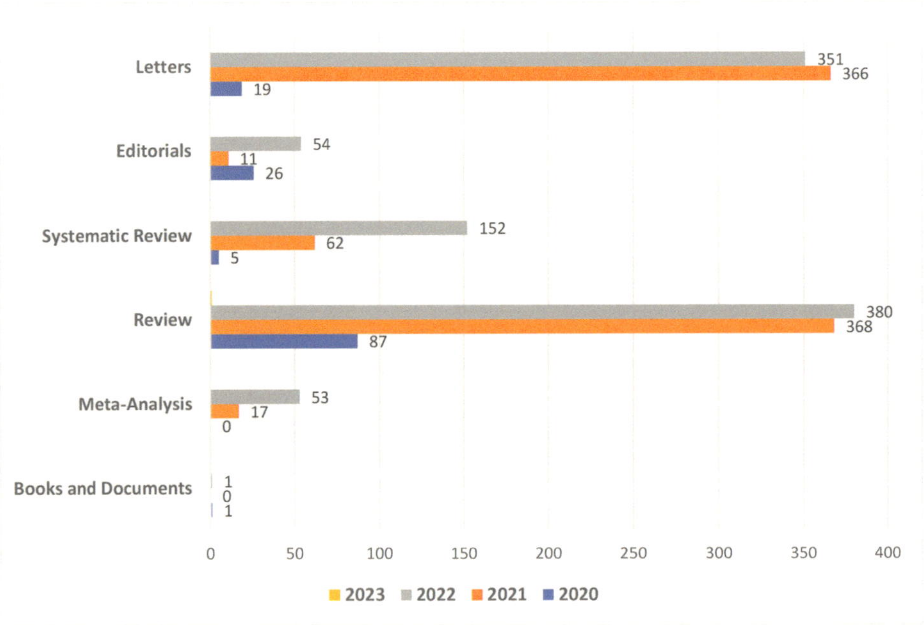

Figure 2.
Research article types on the COVID-19 vaccine development.

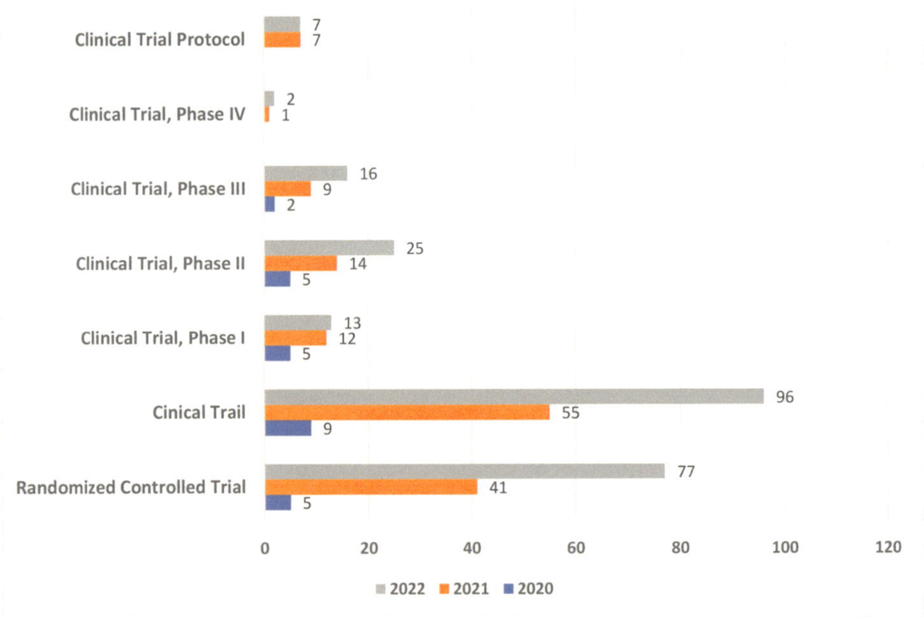

Figure 3.
Research articles on the clinical trials of the COVID-19 vaccine.

number of publications has increased by over 10-fold in 2021 and 2022. This showed the international community's very extensive and focused research efforts toward developing vaccines against this deadly pandemic SARS-CoV-2 virus.

The literature analysis and research publications on PubMed-indexed journals from 2019 to 2022 (**Figure 2**) toward the development of COVID-19 vaccines for the past 3 years of the SARS-CoV-2 pandemic revealed that the majority of publications were Reviews (835 publications) [e.g., see 1, 2, 9, 10], Letters (736 publications) [e.g., see 12–16], Clinical trial-related (401 publications) [e.g., see 4, 17–25], following Systematic reviews (219 publications) [e.g., see 26–30], Editorials (91 publications) [e.g., see 31–35], and Meta-analyses (70 publications) [e.g., see 36–38]. Almost 1200 articles published have associated data. Two books covering COVID-19 vaccines have been published in 2020 [39] and 2022 [40].

Based on the filtration for the clinical trial article category (**Figure 3**), one can see that there are more articles on clinical trials in 2021 than in 2020 and increased by almost 11 times in 2022 compared with 2020. We observed research result publication of clinical trials of phases 1–3 from 2020 to 2022 [4, 17–25] while phase 4 trial results were available in 2021 [41] and 2022 [42, 43].

3. Conclusion

Thus, global research efforts toward the development of COVID-19 vaccines provided state-of-the-art vaccines against the infectious SARS-CoV-2 virus saving millions of lives to date, demonstrating the importance of "deep science" for securing the economy, human health, and life. The current and future development trends dedicated to the development of novel vaccines will require more concentration and multi-institutional collaborative efforts.

Author details

Ibrokhim Y. Abdurakhmonov
Center of Genomics and Bioinformatics, Academy of Sciences of Uzbekistan, Republic of Uzbekistan

*Address all correspondence to: i.y.abdurakhmonov@gmail.com

References

[1] Soleimanpour S, Yaghoubi A. COVID-19 vaccine: Where are we now and where should we go? Expert Review of Vaccines. 2021;**20**(1):23-44. DOI: 10.1080/14760584.2021.1875824

[2] Kaur SP, Gupta V. COVID-19 vaccine: A comprehensive status report. Virus Research. 2020;**288**:198114. DOI: 10.1016/j.virusres.2020.198114

[3] World Health Organization [Internet]. 2021. Available from: https://covid19.trackvaccines.org/agency/who/ [Accessed: October 14, 2022]

[4] Dai L, Gao L, Tao L, Hadinegoro SR, Musaboev M, Ying Z, et al. Efficacy and safety of the RBD-dimer based Covid-19 vaccine ZF2001 in adults. The New England Journal of Medicine. 2022;**386**(22):2097-2111. DOI: 10.1056/NEJMoa2202261

[5] Ayubov MS, Buriev ZT, Mirzakhmedov MK, Yusupov AN, Usmanov DE, Shermatov SE, et al. Profiling of the most reliable mutations from sequenced SARS-CoV-2 genomes scattered in Uzbekistan. PLoS One. 2022;**17**(3):e0266417. DOI: 10.1371/journal.pone.0266417

[6] Abdullaev A, Abdurakhimov A, Mirakbarova Z, Ibragimova S, Tsoy V, Nuriddinov S, et al. Genome sequence diversity of SARS-CoV-2 obtained from clinical samples in Uzbekistan. PLoS One. 2022;**17**(6):e0270314. DOI: 10.1371/journal.pone.0270314

[7] Garib V, Katsamaki S, Turdikulova S, Levitskaya Y, Zahidova N, Bus G, et al. Milk of cow and goat, immunized by recombinant protein vaccine ZF-UZ-VAC2001(Zifivax), contains neutralizing antibodies against SARS-CoV-2 and remains active after standard Milk pasteurization. Frontiers in Nutrition. 2022;**9**:901871. DOI: 10.3389/fnut.2022.901871

[8] Our Word in Data [Internet]. 2021. Available from: https://ourworldindata.org/covid-vaccinations [Accessed: October 14, 2022]

[9] Wibawa T. COVID-19 vaccine research and development: Ethical issues. Tropical Medicine & International Health. 2021;**26**(1):14-19. DOI: 10.1111/tmi.13503

[10] Troiano G, Nardi A. Vaccine hesitancy in the era of COVID-19. Public Health. 2021;**194**:245-251. DOI: 10.1016/j.puhe.2021.02.025

[11] PubMed database [Internet]. 2021. Available from: http://www.ncbi.nlm.nih.gov/pubmed [Accessed: October 12, 2022]

[12] Maurya SP, Das N, Gautam H, Singh R, Das BK. The narrow road to a COVID-19 vaccine. Indian Journal of Pharmacology. 2020;**52**(4):333-334. DOI: 10.4103/ijp.IJP_709_20

[13] Karim SA. COVID-19 vaccine affordability and accessibility. Lancet. 2020;**396**(10246):238. DOI: 10.1016/S0140-6736(20)31540-3

[14] Kane PB, Moyer H, MacPherson A, Papenburg J, Ward BJ, Broomell SB, et al. Expert forecasts of COVID-19 vaccine development timelines. Journal of General Internal Medicine. 2020;**35**(12):3753-3755. DOI: 10.1007/s11606-020-06244-9

[15] Shader RI. COVID-19 vaccine effectiveness. Clinical Therapeutics.

2021;**43**(6):1132-1133. DOI: 10.1016/j.clinthera.2021.04.016

[16] Lacy J, Pavord S, Brown KE. VITT and second doses of Covid-19 vaccine. The New England Journal of Medicine. 2022;**386**(1):95. DOI: 10.1056/NEJMc2118507

[17] Zhu FC, Guan XH, Li YH, Huang JY, Jiang T, Hou LH, et al. Immunogenicity and safety of a recombinant adenovirus type-5-vectored COVID-19 vaccine in healthy adults aged 18 years or older: A randomised, double-blind, placebo-controlled, phase 2 trial. Lancet. 2020;**396**(10249):479-488. DOI: 10.1016/S0140-6736(20)31605-6

[18] Thomas SJ, Moreira ED Jr, Kitchin N, Absalon J, Gurtman A, Lockhart S, et al. Safety and efficacy of the BNT162b2 mRNA Covid-19 vaccine through 6 months. The New England Journal of Medicine. 2021;**385**(19):1761-1773. DOI: 10.1056/NEJMoa2110345

[19] Heath PT, Galiza EP, Baxter DN, Boffito M, Browne D, Burns F, et al. Safety and efficacy of NVX-CoV2373 Covid-19 vaccine. The New England Journal of Medicine. 2021;**385**(13):1172-1183. DOI: 10.1056/NEJMoa2107659

[20] Shinde V, Bhikha S, Hoosain Z, Archary M, Bhorat Q, Fairlie L, et al. Efficacy of NVX-CoV2373 Covid-19 vaccine against the B.1.351 variant. The New England Journal of Medicine. 2021;**384**(20):1899-1909. DOI: 10.1056/NEJMoa2103055

[21] Wu S, Huang J, Zhang Z, Wu J, Zhang J, Hu H, et al. Safety, tolerability, and immunogenicity of an aerosolized adenovirus type-5 vector-based COVID-19 vaccine (Ad5-nCoV) in adults: Preliminary report of an open-label and randomised phase 1 clinical trial. The Lancet Infectious Diseases. 2021;**21**(12):1654-1664. DOI: 10.1016/S1473-3099(21)00396-0

[22] Munro APS, Janani L, Cornelius V, Aley PK, Babbage G, Baxter D, et al. Safety and immunogenicity of seven COVID-19 vaccines as a third dose (booster) following two doses of ChAdOx1 nCov-19 or BNT162b2 in the UK (COV-BOOST): A blinded, multicentre, randomised, controlled, phase 2 trial. Lancet. 2021;**398**(10318):2258-2276. DOI: 10.1016/S0140-6736(21)02717-3

[23] Falsey AR, Sobieszczyk ME, Hirsch I, Sproule S, Robb ML, Corey L, et al. Phase 3 safety and efficacy of AZD1222 (ChAdOx1 nCoV-19) Covid-19 vaccine. The New England Journal of Medicine. 2021;**385**(25):2348-2360. DOI: 10.1056/NEJMoa2105290

[24] Freeman D, Loe BS, Yu LM, Freeman J, Chadwick A, Vaccari C, et al. Effects of different types of written vaccination information on COVID-19 vaccine hesitancy in the UK (OCEANS-III): A single-blind, parallel-group, randomised controlled trial. The Lancet Public Health. 2021;**6**(6):e416-e427. DOI: 10.1016/S2468-2667(21)00096-7

[25] Xia S, Zhang Y, Wang Y, Wang H, Yang Y, Gao GF, et al. Safety and immunogenicity of an inactivated COVID-19 vaccine, BBIBP-CorV, in people younger than 18 years: A randomised, double-blind, controlled, phase 1/2 trial. The Lancet Infectious Diseases. 2022;**22**(2):196-208. DOI: 10.1016/S1473-3099(21)00462-X

[26] Yuan P, Ai P, Liu Y, Ai Z, Wang Y, Cao W, et al. Safety, tolerability, and immunogenicity of COVID-19 vaccines: A systematic review and meta-analysis. medRxiv [Preprint]. 2020; 4:2020.11.03.20224998. DOI: 10.1101/2020.11.03.20224998.

[27] Kaur RJ, Dutta S, Bhardwaj P, Charan J, Dhingra S, Mitra P, et al. Adverse events reported from COVID-19 vaccine trials: A systematic review. Indian Journal of Clinical Biochemistry. 2021;**36**(4):427-439. DOI: 10.1007/s12291-021-00968-z

[28] Sallam M. COVID-19 vaccine hesitancy worldwide: A concise systematic review of vaccine acceptance rates. Vaccines (Basel). 2021;**9**(2):160. DOI: 10.3390/vaccines9020160

[29] Chenchula S, Karunakaran P, Sharma S, Chavan M. Current evidence on efficacy of COVID-19 booster dose vaccination against the omicron variant: A systematic review. Journal of Medical Virology. 2022;**94**(7):2969-2976. DOI: 10.1002/jmv.27697

[30] Venkatesan K, Menon S, Haroon NN. COVID-19 vaccine hesitancy among medical students: A systematic review. Journal of Education Health Promotion. 2022;**11**:218. DOI: 10.4103/jehp.jehp_940_21

[31] Heaton PM. The Covid-19 vaccine-development multiverse. The New England Journal of Medicine. 2020;**383**(20):1986-1988. DOI: 10.1056/NEJMe2025111

[32] Kherabi Y, Fiolet T, Rozencwajg S, Salaün JP, Peiffer-Smadja N. COVID-19 vaccine boosters: What do we know so far? Anaesthesia, Critical Care & Pain Medicine. 2021;**40**(6):100959. DOI: 10.1016/j.accpm.2021.100959

[33] Hauptman M, Vasic J, Krase J. COVID-19 vaccine and biologics: An impending dilemma. Journal of Drugs in Dermatology. 2021;**20**(1):115-114. DOI: 10.36849/JDD.5628

[34] Osama T, Razai MS, Majeed A. Covid-19 vaccine passports: Access, equity, and ethics. BMJ. 2021;**373**:n861. DOI: 10.1136/bmj.n861

[35] Lee ACK, Morling JR. COVID-19 vaccine dilemmas. Public Health. 2022;**202**:10-11. DOI: 10.1016/j.puhe.2021.01.009

[36] Rotshild V, Hirsh-Raccah B, Miskin I, Muszkat M, Matok I. Comparing the clinical efficacy of COVID-19 vaccines: A systematic review and network meta-analysis. Scientific Reports. 2021;**11**(1):22777. DOI: 10.1038/s41598-021-02321-z

[37] Haas JW, Bender FL, Ballou S, Kelley JM, Wilhelm M, Miller FG, et al. Frequency of adverse events in the placebo arms of COVID-19 vaccine trials: A systematic review and meta-analysis. JAMA Network Open. 2022;**5**(1):e2143955. DOI: 10.1001/jamanetworkopen.2021.43955

[38] Au WY, Cheung PP. Effectiveness of heterologous and homologous covid-19 vaccine regimens: Living systematic review with network meta-analysis. BMJ. 2022;**377**:e069989. DOI: 10.1136/bmj-2022-069989

[39] Kahn B, Brown L, Foege W, Gayle H, editors. Framework for Equitable Allocation of COVID-19 Vaccine. Washington (DC): National Academies Press (US); 2020. p. 252. DOI: 10.17226/25917

[40] Aleem A, Nadeem AJ. Coronavirus (COVID-19) Vaccine-Induced Immune Thrombotic Thrombocytopenia (VITT). Treasure Island (FL): StatPearls Publishing; 2022. Available from: https://www.ncbi.nlm.nih.gov/books/NBK570605/ [Accessed: October 12, 2022]

[41] Lazarus R, Baos S, Cappel-Porter H, Carson-Stevens A, Clout M, Culliford L,

et al. Safety and immunogenicity of concomitant administration of COVID-19 vaccines (ChAdOx1 or BNT162b2) with seasonal influenza vaccines in adults in the UK (ComFluCOV): A multicentre, randomised, controlled, phase 4 trial. Lancet. 2021;**398**(10318):2277-2287. DOI: 10.1016/S0140-6736(21)02329-1

[42] Li J, Hou L, Guo X, Jin P, Wu S, Zhu J, et al. Heterologous AD5-nCOV plus CoronaVac versus homologous CoronaVac vaccination: A randomized phase 4 trial. Nature Medicine. 2022;**28**(2):401-409. DOI: 10.1038/s41591-021-01677-z

[43] Costa Clemens SA, Weckx L, Clemens R, Almeida Mendes AV, Ramos Souza A, Silveira MBV, et al. Heterologous versus homologous COVID-19 booster vaccination in previous recipients of two doses of CoronaVac COVID-19 vaccine in Brazil (RHH-001): A phase 4, non-inferiority, single blind, randomised study. Lancet. 2022;**399**(10324):521-529. DOI: 10.1016/S0140-6736(22)00094-0

Section 2

COVID-19 Vaccines and Vaccination

Chapter 2

The COVID-19 Vaccines: The Current Standpoint

Jaeyoung Kim and Nikita Thapa

Abstract

Coronavirus disease 2019 (COVID-19) is a global pandemic that has affected millions of people worldwide. Vaccination seems to be the potent solution to achieve herd immunity and limit viral spread. Various platforms have been utilized to manufacture COVID-19 vaccines such as adenovirus-based vaccines, inactivated virus, DNA-based vaccines, recombinant protein, or mRNA-based vaccines. This chapter covers different viewpoints and the present status of in-use vaccine including the advantages and disadvantages.

Keywords: SARS-CoV-2, vaccine, variant of concerns (VOCs)

1. Introduction

Coronavirus disease 2019 (COVID-19), first reported in Wuhan, China, was declared a pandemic by the World Health Organization (WHO) in March 2020. The WHO confirmed 364,191,494 cases of COVID-19, including 5,631,457 deaths as of January 2022.

Severe acute respiratory syndrome coronavirus 2 (SARS CoV 2), a single-stranded RNA virus, is the causative agent of COVID-19. This virus belongs to the coronavirus family, a group of enveloped viruses that primarily cause respiratory illness. The SARS CoV 2 genome is composed of a 30 kb RNA, five main open reading frames, four primary structural proteins—spikes (S), envelopes (E), membranes (M), and nucleocapsids (N), all of which trigger immunological responses (**Figure 1**). The entry of virus into host is via angiotensin-converting enzyme 2 (ACE2) receptor-mediated attachment of the S protein to the host cell. The internalization of viral S protein and subsequent integration into the host cell are mediated by the serine protease of the host cell, transmembrane serine protease 2 [1].

With the increasing global prevalence of COVID-19 cases, the development of an effective vaccine is imperative to contain the pandemic. Vaccinations have the capability to generate herd immunity in societies, which can reduce disease occurrence, transmission, and the social and economic detrimental impact of the disease. No specific antiviral treatment is currently available for public use. However, since the SARS CoV 2 genomic sequence was identified, >100 vaccine studies have been performed, ~50 of which have reached human experimentation, and several vaccines

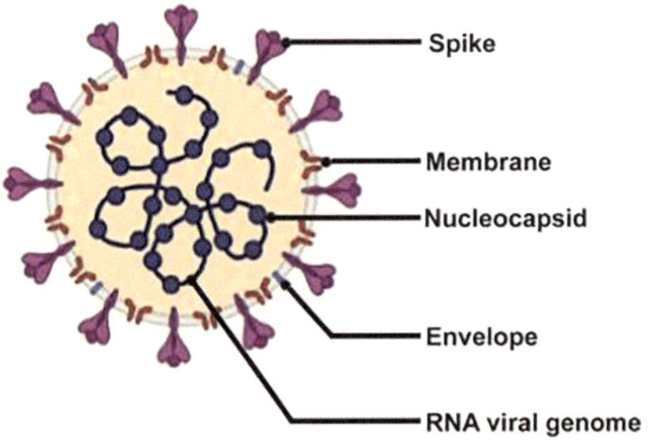

Figure 1.
Diagrammatic view of severe acute respiratory syndrome coronavirus 2. The virus is principally composed of four structural proteins spike, envelope, membrane, and nucleocapsid.

are currently being administered to certain sections of the population (ourworldindata.org/covid vaccinations). At present, only few numbers of vaccines have received FDA approval for public use.

2. COVID-19 vaccines: Platform

Vaccinations are the only safest and most cost-effective strategy for preventing COVID-19 disease transmission in public. The intent behind vaccine development is to induce a primary immune response by delivering altered or weakened antigens that normally cause disease, allowing the host to form immunological memory without getting infected naturally.

The most critical step in the development of vaccines is selecting the protective and immunogenic epitope. The primary targets to induce humoral immune response are S and N proteins of coronavirus. The receptor binding domain (RBD) of the S protein, followed by the N protein, is the primary antigenic target of SARS-CoV-2 for neutralizing human IgM, IgG, and IgA [2]. Long-term protection depends on the persistence of vaccine-induced antibodies above protective thresholds and/or the maintenance of immunological memory cells capable of quick and effective reactivation following subsequent exposure [3].

To combat this pandemic, there are chances that the world will certainly require more than a single vaccine type or single antigen/epitope to induce an immunological response that should cater to the need for broad target population coverage, high production volume, and storage and transportation requirements in addition to vaccine safety and effectiveness.

For the development of the COVID-19 vaccine, several vaccination platforms have been investigated, each with its own set of benefits and drawbacks (**Table 1** shows the comparative chart of advantages and disadvantages of vaccines based on different platforms). The ongoing vaccine development trial involves classical molecular strategies that are based upon inactivated, modified live or attenuated virus, single peptides, or viral vectors (**Figure 2**) [4].

Vaccine Types	Advantages	Disadvantages
Adenoviral vector vaccines	• Direct production of antigen in the cell of interest • Multiple epitopes can be included • Scalable production globally • Most immunogenic viral vectors	• Pre-existing anti-adenovirus immunity and potential adverse events • Potentially cause dangerous blood clots • Lack of strong, long-lasting immunity after single dose
DNA vaccines	• Stimulation of both humoral and cell-mediated immunity • Efficient large-scale, low-cost, production and high storage Stability	• Need delivery agent to be translocated into the nucleus • Low immune response • Only been licensed for use in veterinary medicine
RNA vaccines	• Ease and rapidity of assembling new mRNA sequences into existing vaccine formulations • Nontoxic and non-immunogenic • No risk of integration with the host cell genome	• Rare, severe anaphylactic reactions • Long-term immunity issue • Expensive to manufacture
Protein Subunit vaccines	• Easy to produce at large-scale (cost-efficient). • Can be produced in different expression systems • Well-defined composition	• Expression of a fragment of the protein • Usually elicits weak immune responses
Whole Virus Vaccines	• Stimulation of protective immune response • Induce both cellular and humoral immune response	• Chances of viral mutations inducing increases in toxicity and adverse reactions post vaccination
Extracellular vesicle (EV)-based vaccines	• Excellent carriers for viral antigens; present the antigens in their native state • Can pass through the blood–brain barrier	• Production and scalability are difficult • Characterization of immune responses for each disease needs further research

Table 1.
Advantages and disadvantages of available vaccine approach.

2.1 Whole virus vaccines

The whole virus vaccine consists of a weakened form of SARS-CoV-2, which has been attenuated or inactivated so that without causing any harmful effect it can induce a protective immune response. Inactivated vaccines can only induce humoral immune responses to SARS-CoV-2, whereas live-activated vaccines can stimulate both cellular and humoral immune responses [5].

2.2 Nucleic-acid-based vaccine

The nucleic-acid-based vaccine uses the genetic material of the pathogen as an active component of the vaccine. Based on the type of genetic material, it could be DNA or mRNA-based vaccines where RNA vaccine could be further subdivided

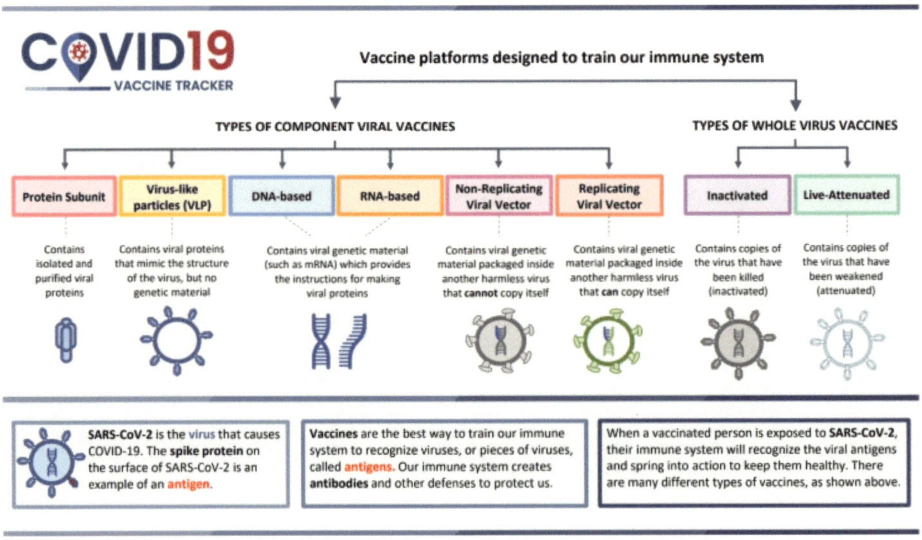

Figure 2.
Current vaccine platform, designed to manufacture vaccine against COVID-19. Taken from https://covid19.trackvaccines.org/vaccine-types/.

into mRNA vaccine. Both vaccination platforms can elicit primarily B- and T-cell responses, but with different risk profiles. In the current scenario of the COVID-19 pandemic, genetic material of SARS-CoV-2 is used to induce immune response [4].

2.3 Viral vector vaccines

Viral vector vaccines that are designed against SARS-Cov-2 use modified viral vectors that carry gene encoding of spike proteins. As a vector, these vaccines use modified versions of several viruses. Several different types of viruses have been utilized as vectors, the most frequently used are adenoviruses [5].

2.4 Protein subunit vaccines

Protein subunit vaccines are made of one or more purified antigens from the viruses or bacteria of interest that are capable of eliciting the immune response and imparting a protective response. In terms of SARS Cov-2, these are spike proteins (S), which have been produced in vitro. Two common forms of protein subunit vaccines are polysaccharide and conjugate vaccines against SARS-CoV-2. Polysaccharide vaccines comprise SARS-CoV-2 cell wall polysaccharides, whereas conjugate candidates are coupled to a polysaccharide chain with a carrier protein to generate a boost in the immune system response [4].

2.5 Virus-like particles (VLPs)

Virus-like particles (VLPs) are a type of protein vaccines that are made up of nanoparticles that look like viruses. VLPs are composed of some or all the proteins that make up the viral capsid, rather than a single protein. They resemble live attenuated or inactivated vaccines in that they can elicit strong cellular and humoral immune responses while posing no risk of reversion since they lack the virus's genetic material [6].

2.6 Exosome-based vaccines

Exosomes are lipid bilayer coated extracellular vesicles secreted by a variety of cells. Their key role is to function in intercellular communication, and they have been reported to load RNA, DNA, and proteins in between cells. The key features of EV-based vaccines, including their ability to induce poor immunogenicity, mean EVs can be safely and efficiently used in vaccine development. The ability of EVs to preserve naïve antigen conformation and access to all organs via bodily fluids gives an added advantage compared with other delivery agents, such as lipid-based nanoparticles (LNPs) or viral vectors. Unlike other platforms, these vaccines are in the very preliminary phase of vaccine development. Although many companies including Capricor Therapeutics have shown positive preclinical results, none of them has still managed to enter phase 1 clinical trials [7].

3. COVID-19 vaccines: Current status

The US Food and Drug Administration (FDA) has approved three COVID-19 vaccines for emergency use: two messenger RNA-based vaccines (Pfizer and Moderna) and one adenoviral vector vaccine (Janssen). In case of a public health emergency, unlicensed drugs and vaccines are given emergency use authorization (EUA). Currently, as per the WHO data, there are 10 vaccines that have been granted for Emergency Use Listing (EUL) as of April 25, 2022 [8] (**Table 2**). Two vaccines (Moderna and Janssen) have completed phase 4 clinical trials successfully. At present, 153 COVID-19 candidates are in clinical trials and 196 candidates are in preclinical research worldwide [9]. Below is a brief description of three FDA-approved vaccines for COVID-19.

3.1 Pfizer–BioNTech (BNT162b2)

BNT162b2 is a lipid nanoparticle (LNP)-formulated, nucleoside-modified RNA vaccine that encodes the full-length SARS-CoV-2 spike (S) protein, modified by two proline mutations to ensure an antigenically optimal pre-fusion conformation that mimics the intact virus to trigger virus-neutralizing antibodies. This vaccine showed good safety and efficacy, and after about 12 days of vaccination, this vaccine has reportedly shown a reduction in the risk of SARS-CoV-2 infection. By April 2022, among all available vaccines, the Pfizer vaccine has shown to exhibit the highest efficacy of 95% and is WHO-approved in 103 countries. The minor side effects that were reported for this vaccine are pain at the injection site, fatigue, headache, muscle and joint pain, chills, fever, and diarrhea. While rare side effects include pericarditis, arrhythmia, deep-vein thrombosis, pulmonary embolism, myocardial infarction, intracranial hemorrhage, and thrombocytopenia [10].

3.2 mRNA-1273 Moderna

Moderna's mRNA vaccine is a lipid nanoparticle-encapsulated nucleoside-modified messenger RNA (mRNA)-based vaccine. It encodes the SARS-CoV-2

Vaccine Name	Vaccine Type	Approval Status/ Authorization	Clinical Trials
Novavax Nuvaxovid	Protein Subunit	Approved in 37 countries	15 trials in 12 countries
Serum Institute of India COVOVAX (Novavax formulation)	Protein Subunit	Approved in 4 countries	2 trials in 1 country
Moderna Spikevax	RNA	Approved in 85 countries	60 trials in 22 countries
Pfizer/BioNTech Comirnaty	RNA	Approved in 144 countries	73 trials in 26 countries
Janssen (Johnson & Johnson) Ad26.COV2.S	Non-Replicating Viral Vector	Approved in 111 countries	20 trials in 22 countries
Oxford/AstraZeneca Vaxzevria	Non-Replicating Viral Vector	Approved in 138 countries	62 trials in 30 countries
Serum Institute of India Covishield (Oxford/ AstraZeneca)	Non-Replicating Viral Vector	Approved in 47 countries	2 trials in 1 country
Bharat Biotech Covaxin	Inactivated	Approved in 14 countries	10 trials in 2 countries
Sinopharm (Beijing) Covilo	Inactivated	Approved in 91 countries	26 trials in 12 countries
Sinovac CoronaVac	Inactivated	Approved in 55 countries	37 trials in 9 countries

Table 2.
WHO list of vaccines approved for emergency use listing (EUL).

full-length spike protein that has been prefusion stabilized. This spike glycoprotein regulates the adhesion to host cells. As a result, it is required for viral entry and hence serves as the primary target for the vaccine. The vaccine causes a strong binding and neutralizing response. Like the Pfizer vaccine, this is among those first vaccines that received EUA in December 2020. This vaccine has shown efficacy of 94% and is WHO-approved in 76 countries. The most common side effects are headache, injection site pain, fatigue, muscle pain, and chills. Rare side effects include nausea, vomiting, myocarditis, pericarditis, angioedema, and anaphylaxis [11].

3.3 Janssen vaccine/Ad26.COV2.S

Janssen's Ad26.COV2 S vaccine is a recombinant human adenovirus type 26 that carries the full-length SARS-CoV-2 S protein and generates an antibody response against the SARS-CoV-2 infection. The Janssen vaccine is based on the deletion of the E1 gene and the replacement of it with the spike gene in inactivated adenoviruses. The adjuvant properties, scalability, and broad tissue tropism of adenoviral vectors are advantages. This vaccine shows an efficacy of 66.9%, and WHO has approved it in 75 countries. Like other vaccines, common localized side effects reported are pain at the inoculation site and systemic signs such as fever, headache, myalgia, or nausea [12]. **Table 3** depicts the most used COVID-19 vaccine worldwide with the efficacy, storage temperature, and route of administration.

As per the World database (ourworldindata.org/covid-vaccinations), COVID-19 vaccination has been administered to 65.4% of the world's population (April,2022).

S. No.	Vaccine/ Manufacturer	Efficacy	Storage temperature	Route
1.	Pfizer BioNTech	95.3%	−80 degrees C to −60 degrees C	Intra-muscular
2.	AstraZeneca	63.09%	+2 degrees C to +8 degrees C	Intra-muscular
3.	Sputnik-V	91.6%	+2 degrees C to +8 degrees C (Dry form) −18.5 degree C (Liquid form)	Intra-muscular
4.	Moderna	94.1%	+2 degrees C to +8 degrees C (for 30 days) -50 degrees C to −15 degrees C	Intra-muscular
5.	Janssen/Johnson	66.3%	+2 degrees C to +8 degrees C	Intra-muscular
6.	Covaxin	78%	+2 degrees C to +8 degrees C	Intra-muscular

Table 3.
List of key features of commonly used COVID-19 vaccines with efficacy.

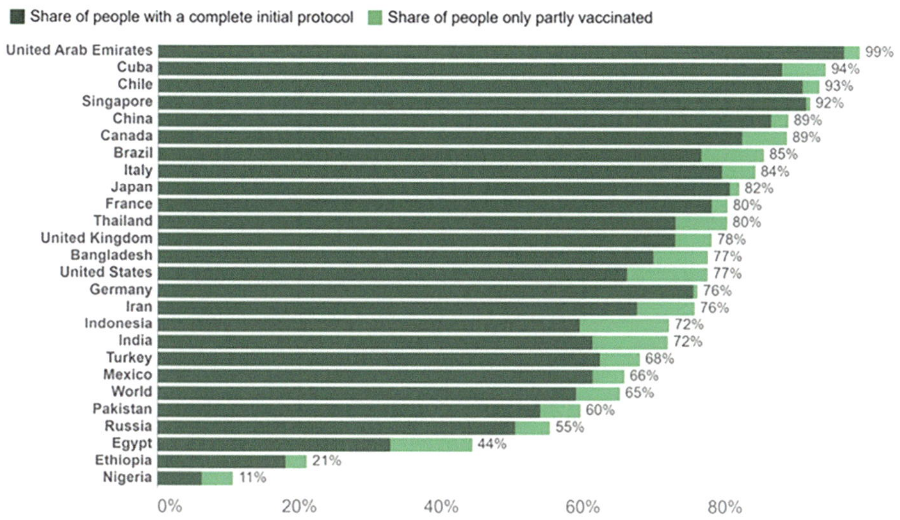

Figure 3.
Graphical representation of people vaccinated against COVID-19 for some countries as of Apr 27, 2022. Taken from https://ourworldindata.org/covid-vaccinations.

Globally, 11.6 billion doses have been rolled out, with 9.82 million doses being given out every day. In low-income countries, just 15.7% of people have had at least one dose. **Figure 3** shows a graphical representation of people in several nations who have been vaccinated against COVID-19.

4. Limitations of vaccines

Regardless of multiple attempts of developing vaccines for SARS-CoV-2, the chances of complete eradication of diseases still face various challenges, which may arise due to varied levels of efficacy or preexisting immunity or limited accessibility. Thus, an effective vaccine needs to overcome multiple obstacles as stated below:

4.1 Long-term outcome

Since efficacy was determined based on short-term evidence, especially when other vaccines have shown efficacy declining with time. The antibody induction by of Moderna vaccine remained high among all age groups and lasted for 6 months after the second dose. After 6 months, there has been no further information [13]. Furthermore, current trials have revealed no long-term problems.

4.2 Preexisting immunity

Currently available SARS CoV 2 vaccines (AstraZeneca/Janssen) are based on the classical approach of viral vectors, particularly adenoviruses. Although adenovirus-based vaccines are well characterized, they are limited by preexisting immunity of the virus vector employed in the vaccine design, which may restrict the immune response against COVID-19 antigens, thereby decreasing their efficacy [14].

4.3 Antibody-dependent enhancement (ADE)

Another point of concern is the risk of reinfection with emerging viruses in the community due to a lack of long-lasting immunity. Multiple immunizations with such viral vectors, if not effective, could lead to a more complicated form of the disease, such as antibody-dependent enhancement (ADE), increasing the disease burden in a vaccinated person [15].

4.4 Variant protection

New variants of SARS-CoV-2 have the potential to complicate the effectiveness of current vaccines. In the United Kingdom, ChAdOx1 demonstrated 75% protection against one variant named B.1.1.7 (including asymptomatic infection). However, the AstraZeneca vaccine showed only 10% protection against the B.1.351 variant in a young population with a median age of 30 in South Africa, hence their AstraZeneca roll-out was ceased [16]. Thus, an effective approach for vaccine development is required, which can also overcome the issue of variant of concerns (VOCs).

4.5 Age groups

Age is also one of the crucial factors to check the effectiveness of vaccination. In all age groups and persons with comorbidities, further evaluation of the efficacy of all vaccines is necessary. Individuals above the age of 16 took part in Pfizer's vaccine trials. Individuals 18 years and older were included in the Moderna, Oxford/AstraZeneca, and Janssen trials. At this time, Oxford/AstraZeneca appears to be more tolerated in older adults than in younger adults, and it has similar immunogenicity in all age groups following a booster dosage [17].

5. Future perspectives of vaccine development

Active immunization represents the most effective technique for combating the current COVID-19 pandemic and saving millions of lives around the world. The currently approved vaccines have been shown to reduce both mortality and the incidence of severe COVID-19 infection, and they are now a critical weapon in the fight against SARS-CoV-2. The rising cases of variant of concerns (VOCs), on the other hand, continue to pose a threat to vaccine-induced immune protection, emphasizing the need for multi-coronavirus vaccine platforms capable of inducing a long-lasting protective immune response.

The key strategy for combating the COVID-19 pandemic is to develop vaccines that can induce long-lasting immunity and protect against circulating SARS-CoV-2 variants. Ongoing trials for SARS CoV 2 vaccine construction are based on the principle of eliciting neutralizing antibodies (Nabs) against the S protein, thereby interfering with viral receptor binding. To date, research associated with COVID-19 vaccine development has focused primarily on antibody titers and the ability of antibodies to neutralize viral particles [18].

But, with the accumulating evidence of potential roles of more conserved non-spike viral antigens, such as nucleocapsid (N) proteins, which could bring a major victory in the battle against COVID-19 VOCs and can also overcome the existing issue of providing long-lasting immunity. Immunologically, a vaccine that targets the mutation-prone S protein, as well as the more stable and conserved N, is required to surmount the immune escape characteristics exhibited by SARS CoV 2 variants [19].

The rapid development of the COVID-19 vaccine within such a short life span represents a remarkable landmark in the history of antiviral vaccine development. This progress has also given hope to the development of the long-time pending dream of developing an HIV vaccine. Many pharmaceuticals such as Moderna and Pfizer are trying to develop the HIV vaccine for past decades but have been unsuccessful in its clinical translation. Thanks to SARS CoV-2, such rapid progression and successful results of the COVID-19 vaccine made decade long dream of HIV vaccine development possible now and such vaccine candidates are currently under clinical trials.

6. Conclusion

With the purpose of making world COVID free, available vaccines possess many drawbacks that need to be addressed. Besides following the proper implementation of preventive measures, we need to focus on all the major vaccination strategies to achieve a successful outcome. It is imperative to consider multiple antigens/multi epitope vaccine to achieve long-term immunity and protection against a variant of concerns (VOCs). However, even though there are still numerous hurdles and unanswered concerns, the tremendous advances in COVID-19 vaccine research have given the world hope that this disease can be eradicated.

Author details

Jaeyoung Kim* and Nikita Thapa
CK-Exogene, Inc., Seongnam, Gyeonggi-do, Republic of Korea

*Address all correspondence to: caput@naver.com

References

[1] Mousavizadeh L, Ghasemi S. Genotype and phenotype of COVID-19: Their roles in pathogenesis. Journal of Microbiology, Immunology, and Infection. 2021;**54**:159-163. DOI: 10.1016/j.jmii.2020.03.022

[2] Francica JRFB, Foulds KE, Noe AT, Werner AP, Moore IN, et al. Protective antibodies elicited by SARS-CoV-2 spike protein vaccination are boosted in the lung after challenge in nonhuman primates. Science Translational Medicine. 2021;**13**:eabi4547. DOI:10.1126/scitranslmed.abi4547

[3] Sadarangani M, Marchant A, Kollmann TR. Immunological mechanisms of vaccine-induced protection against COVID-19 in humans. Nature Reviews. Immunology. 2021;**21**:475-484. DOI: 10.1016/j.medcle.2021.11.005

[4] Tregoning JS, Brown ES, Cheeseman HM, et al. Vaccines for COVID-19. Clinical and Experimental Immunology. 2020;**202**:162-192. DOI: 10.1111/cei.13517

[5] Lundstrom K. Viral vectors for COVID-19 vaccine development. Viruses. 2021;**13**:317. DOI: 10.3390/v13020317

[6] Syomin B, Ilyin Y. Virus-like particles as an instrument of vaccine production. Molecular Biology. 2019;**53**:323-334. DOI: 10.1134/S0026893319030154

[7] Yoo KH, Thapa N, Kim BJ, et al. Possibility of exosome-based coronavirus disease 2019 vaccine (review). Molecular Medicine Reports. 2021;**25**:26. DOI: 10.3892/mmr.2021.12542

[8] FDA Emergency Use Authorization. Available online: https://www.fda.gov.ph/list-of-fda-issued-emergency-use-authorization. [Accessed: May 2, 2022]

[9] Gavi The COVID-19 Vaccine Race—Weekly Update. Available online: https://www.gavi.org/vaccineswork/covid-19-vaccine-race?gclid=Cj0KCQjw8eOLBhC1ARIsAOzx5cEoa2VnSPnys3WznKcdeff8JBByVvOjPuCNkXg8P4Gcy0nsLU8xJ5QaAuRwEALw_wcB. [Accessed: April 28, 2022]

[10] Menni C, Klaser K, May A, Polidori L, Capdevila J, Louca P, et al. Vaccine side-effects and SARS-CoV-2 infection after vaccination in users of the COVID symptom study app in the UK: A prospective observational study. The Lancet Infectious Diseases. 2021;**21**:939-949. DOI: 10.1016/S1473-3099(21)00224-3

[11] Hiller N, Goldberg SN, Cohen-Cymberknoh M, Vainstein V, Simanovsky N. Lymphadenopathy associated with the COVID-19 vaccine. Cureus. 2021;**13**:13524. DOI: 10.7759/cureus.13524

[12] Sadoff J, Gray G, Vandebosch A, et al. Safety and efficacy of single-dose Ad26.COV2.S vaccine against Covid-19. The New England Journal of Medicine. 2021;**384**:2187-2201. DOI: 10.1056/NEJMoa2101544

[13] Doria-Rose N, Suthar MS, Makowski M, et al. Antibody persistence through 6 months after the second dose of mRNA-1273 vaccine for Covid-19. The New England Journal of Medicine. 2021;**384**:2259-2261. DOI: 10.1056/NEJMc2103916

[14] Ghaebi M, Osali A, Valizadeh H, Roshangar L, Ahmadi M. Vaccine development and therapeutic design for

2019 nCoV/SARS CoV 2: Challenges and chances. Journal of Cellular Physiology. 2020;**235**:9098-9109. DOI: 10.1002/jcp.29771

[15] Arvin AM, Fink K, Schmid MA, Cathcart A, Spreafico R, Havenar Daughton C, et al. A perspective on potential antibody dependent enhancement of SARS CoV 2. Nature. 2020;**584**(353):363. DOI: 10.1038/s41586-020-2538-8

[16] Gupta RK. Will SARS-CoV-2 variants of concern affect the promise of vaccines? Nature Reviews. Immunology. 2021;**21**:340-341. DOI: 10.1038/s41577-021-00556-5

[17] Ramasamy MN, Minassian AM, Ewer KJ, et al. Safety and immunogenicity of ChAdOx1 nCoV-19 vaccine administered in a prime-boost regimen in young and old adults (COV002): A single-blind, randomised, controlled, phase 2/3 trial. The Lancet. 2020;**396**:1979-1993. DOI: 10.1016/S0140-6736(20)32466-1

[18] Garcia Beltran WF, Lam EC, Astudillo MG, Yang D, Miller TE, Feldman J, et al. COVID 19 neutralizing antibodies predict disease severity and survival. Cell. 2021;**184**(476):488. DOI: 10.1101/2020.10.15.20213512

[19] Garcia Beltran WF, Lam EC, St Denis K, Nitido AD, Garcia ZH, Hauser BM, et al. Multiple SARS CoV 2 variants escape neutralization by vaccine induced humoral immunity. Cell. 2021;**184**(2372):2383. DOI: 10.1016/j.cell.2021.03.013

Chapter 3

ZF2001, A Protein Subunit Vaccines against SARS-CoV-2

Fangwu Chen and Gao Ya

Abstract

Anhui Zhifei Longcom 's Zifivax, also known as ZF2001 (ZF-UZ-VAC-2001) is a protein subunit vaccine using a dimeric form of the receptor-binding domain (RBD) as the antigen, a harmless piece of the SARS-Cov-2 virus. As of June, 2022, over 300 million doses of Zifivax have been vaccinated with localized production in China base and Tashkent, Uzbekistan. At present, the severe acute respiratory syndrome coronavirus 2 (SARS-Cov-2) is constantly mutating and evolving, and the coronavirus disease 2019 (COVID-19) epidemic is seriously threatening human health. Vaccination is the most effective and economical method to prevent and control the COVID-19 pandemic. Research institutions and companies around the world are employing various techniques to develop COVID-19 vaccines. According to the preparation technology, COVID-19 vaccines can be classified as inactivated virus vaccines, live attenuated vaccines, mRNA vaccines, DNA vaccines, viral vector vaccines, virus-like particle vaccines and protein subunit vaccines. Among these, viral protein subunit vaccines based on in vitro production of key viral proteins or peptides from bacterial, yeast, insect or mammalian cells have been drawing attention owing to their advantages of high safety and effectiveness, low cost of production, storage and transportation. Givrn this, this study reviewed the research and development status of ZF2001, as a reference for the development of protein subunit vaccines against SARS-Cov-2.

Keywords: SARS-Cov-2, COVID-19, protein subunit vaccine, R and D principle, research progress

1. Introduction

The coronavirus disease 2019 (COVID-19) is an acute respiratory infectious disease caused by severe acute respiratory syndrome coronavirus 2 (SARS-Cov-2). As of April 8, 2022, COVID-19 has spread to 227 countries, causing 490 million infections and 6.17 million deaths [1]. The raging COVID-19 has seriously affected the global economy and public health. As the most effective and economical means to prevent and control COVID-19, COVID-19 vaccines have been attracting much attention, especially their R and D progress. According to the preparation technology, COVID-19 vaccines can be classified as inactivated virus vaccines, live attenuated vaccines, mRNA vaccines, DNA vaccines, viral vector vaccines, virus-like particle vaccines and protein subunit vaccines [2, 3]. Among these, protein subunit vaccines based on *in vitro* production of key viral proteins or peptides from bacterial, yeast, insect or mammalian cells has been drawing attention because they: (1) contain no viral genetic material and are thus safer than inactivated vaccines; (2) do not feed viruses and can be produced in a production workshop of lower biosafety level; (3) use transgenic technology to achieve high yield and high purity expression of antigens and facilitate large-scale production; and (4) are easy to store and transport [4]. As of April 9, 2022, a total of 36 COVID-19 vaccines have been formally approved by the government's public health department, including 14 types of protein subunit vaccines [5]. In view of this, this research studies the research and development status of some marketed SARS-CoV-2 protein subunit vaccines based on domestic and foreign scientific literature and clinical data, and summarizes its research and development principles and clinical effects, to provide a reference for the research and development of SARS-CoV-2 protein subunit vaccine.

2. R and D principles of SARS-CoV-2 protein subunit vaccine

SARS-CoV-2 is an enveloped, positive-sense, single-stranded RNA virus that encodes 16 non-structural proteins, 9 accessory proteins, and 4 major structural proteins. Among them, the structural proteins are envelope protein (E), membrane protein (M), nucleocapsid protein (N) and spike protein (S) [6]. The S protein present in the viral envelope as a homologous trimer consists of two functional subunits, S1 and S2 (see **Figure 1**). The S1 subunit contains a receptor binding domain (RBD), which recognizes the receptor-angiotensin-converting enzyme 2 (ACE2) on host cells [7]. The S2 subunit contains fusion peptide (FP), junction region (CR), heptad repeat (HR), central helix (CH), etc., to fuse the membranes of viruses and host cells. When the S1 subunit binds to the ACE2 on host cells, the host protease recognizes and cleaves the S1/S2 cleavage site, the S1 subunit dissociates to fuse the membranes of FP that protrude after the conformational changes of the S2 subunit. Previous studies

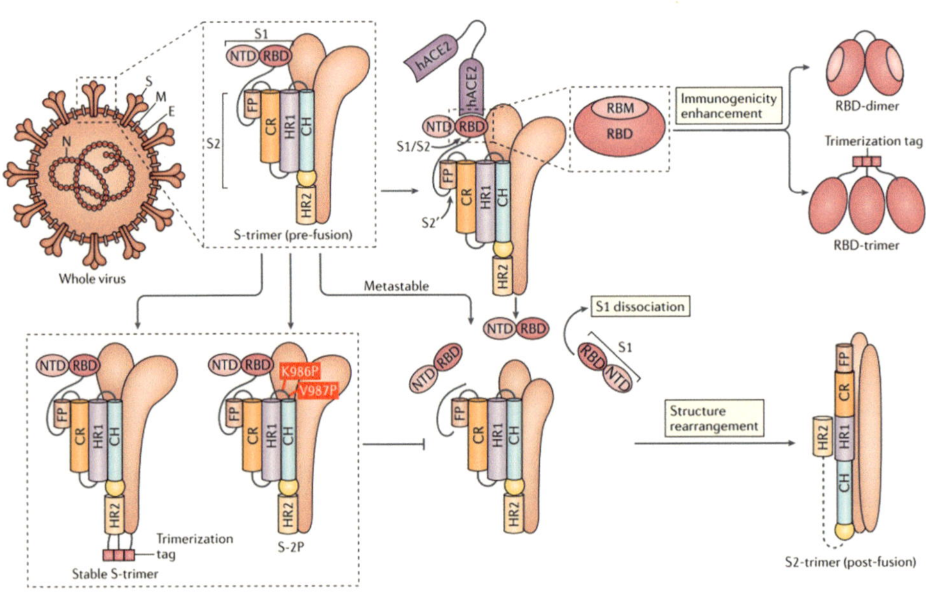

Figure 1.
Main targets for R and D of COVID-19 vaccine [6].

have shown that the RBD region of the S protein of SARS-CoV-2 is immunogenic and is the target of 90% neutralizing antibodies in immunosera [8]. Therefore, the S protein of SARS-CoV-2 has become the main target for the R and D of vaccines.

3. SARS-CoV-2 protein subunit vaccines produced based on RBD

RBD is one of the high-profile vaccine targets, while low immunogenicity limits its application in the vaccine. Adding antigen size, multimerization, or intensive antigen presentation in particles may enhance the immunogenicity of RBD subunit vaccine.

The research team of Gao Fu and Dai Lianpan from the Institute of Microbiology, Chinese Academy of Sciences, found in a study of RBD against MERS-coronavirus that disulfide-linked RBD dimers can induce higher neutralizing antibodies than traditional monomers. To further improve the stability and homogeneity of the dimeric antigen, the team optimized the dimeric protein structure and obtained tandem repeated RBD single-chain dimers. This tandem repeat single-stranded dimer has a single expression form, does not contain exogenous sequences, can maintain high vaccine potency, and is suitable for the R and D of COVID-19 and SARS-CoV-2 vaccines [9]. Based on this design strategy, Anhui Zhifei Longcom Biopharmaceutical Co., Ltd. and the Institute of Microbiology, Chinese Academy of Sciences jointly developed and produced the SARS-CoV-2 protein subunit vaccine ZF2001. In 2020, together with the Center of Advance Technology under the Ministry of Innovative Development of Uzbekistan, the multi-center international Phase 3 clinical trials were launched, data showed that the short-term and long-term protective efficacy against COVID-19 of any severity were 81.4% and 75.7%, respectively, that against Alpha variant was 92.7% and 88.3%, respectively, and that against Delta variant were 81.4% and 76.1%, respectively after three doses of ZF2001 in people over 18 years. This protective efficacy is higher than the WHO-preferred SARS-CoV-2 vaccine standard (70%) [10]. The sera of subjects vaccinated with three doses of inactivated vaccine or ZF2001 were tested by the pseudovirus cross-neutralization test, among which 62.5% sera of subjects vaccinated with inactivated vaccine were found to be positive for the Omicron variant neutralizing antibody while 100% sera of subjects vaccinated with ZF2001 (0, 1 and 5 months dose schedule) were found to be positive for Omicron variant neutralizing antibody [11]. By testing the neutralizing antibody titer, it was found that the titer of Omicron variant was reduced by 5.1-fold in the inactivated vaccine group and only 3-fold in the ZF2001 (0, 1 and 5 months dose schedule) group compared with the wild-type strain [11]. Sunney Xie's team at Peking University showed that after two doses of inactivated vaccine, booster vaccination with ZF2001 induced a higher humoral immune response than with inactivated vaccine (CoronaVac) [12]. Based on the safety and efficacy of ZF2001, ZF2001 was approved for conditional marketing by the National Medical Products Administration on March 2, 2022, becoming the first domestic recombinant SARS-CoV-2 protein vaccine approved for conditional marketing, and will be used as a sequential vaccination to booster the protective effect of the existing vaccine.

4. Summary and outlook

Although it takes a long time to construct and screen engineered cell lines/strains with high expression of antigens in the early stage of the production of protein subunit vaccines, these vaccines have the advantages of high safety and immunogenicity, low production and transportation costs, which can meet the needs of low- and middle-income countries. In addition, COVID-19 protein subunit vaccines can be used as heterologous booster immunizations to trigger more ideal and long-lasting immune responses. Currently, multiple research teams and companies are actively developing COVID-19 protein subunit vaccines.

In order to develop a multivalent vaccine rapidly adapted to SARS-Cov-2 dominant variants, Gao Fu's research team designed prototype-Beta and Delta-Omicron chimeric protein vaccines based on the WT homologous RBD dimer protein vaccine. Animal experiments have shown that the two-protein chimeric vaccine can stimulate a broader spectrum of antibody responses and protective effects. The Delta-Omicron chimeric protein vaccine provided better protection during the challenge test with Delta and Omicron variants [13]. At present, Zhifei Longcom has completed the construction of a cell bank for the Delta-Omicron chimeric protein vaccine.

Currently, billions of people worldwide have not been vaccinated with COVID-19 vaccines. Inequalities in vaccine access may lead to the emergence of more infectious variants. Therefore, it is necessary to continue the development of COVID-19 vaccines from multiple routes.

Author details

Fangwu Chen[1,2*] and Gao Ya[1,2]

1 Anhui Zhifei Longcom Biopharmaceutical Co., Ltd., Anhui, People's Republic of China

2 Chongqing Zhifei Biological Products Co., Ltd., Chongqing, China

*Address all correspondence to: chenfangwu@zhifeishengwu.com

References

[1] WHO. WHO Coronavirus (COVID-19) Dashboard [EB/OL]. (2022-04-08, 2022-04-18]. https://covid19.who.int/

[2] Fathizadeh H, Afshar S, Masoudi MR, et al. SARS-CoV-2 (Covid-19) vaccines structure, mechanisms and effectiveness: A review. International Journal of Biological Macromolecules. 2021;**188**: 740-750

[3] Hadj HI. Covid-19 vaccines and variants of concern: A review. Reviews in Medical Virology. Jul 2022;**32**(4):e2313

[4] Yadav T, Srivastava N, Mishra G, et al. Recombinant vaccines for COVID-19. Human Vaccine Immunotherapeutics. 2020;**16**:2905-2912

[5] COVID-19 Vaccine Tracker. https://covid19.trackvaccines.org/

[6] Dai L, Gao GF. Viral targets for vaccines against COVID-19. Nature Reviews. Immunology. 2021;**21**:73-82

[7] Lan J, Ge J, Yu J, Shan S, et al. Structure of the SARS-CoV-2 spike receptor-binding domain bound to the ACE2 receptor. Nature. 2020;**581**:215-220

[8] Piccoli L, Park YJ, Tortorici MA, et al. Mapping neutralizing and immunodominant sites on the SARS-CoV-2 spike receptor-binding domain by structure-guided high-resolution Serology. Cell. 2020;**183**(4):1024-1042

[9] Dai L, Zheng T, Xu K, et al. A universal design of btacoronavirus vaccines against COVID-19, MERS, and SARS. Cell. 2020;**182**:722-733

[10] Dai L, Gao L, Tao L, et al. Efficacy and safety of the RBD-dimer-based COVID-19 vaccine ZF2001 in adults. The New England Journal of Medicine. 2022;**386**(22):2097-2111

[11] Zhao X, Li D, Ruan W, et al. Effects of a prolonged booster interval on neutralization of Omicron variant. The New England Journal of Medicine. 2022;**386**(9):894-896

[12] Cao Y, Hao X, Wang X, et al. Humoral immunogenicity and reactogenicity of CoronaVac or ZF2001 booster after two doses of inactivated vaccine. Cell Research. 2022;**32**(1):107-109

[13] Xu K, Gao P, Liu S, et al. Protective prototype-Beta and Delta-Omicron chimeric RBD-dimer vaccines against SARS-CoV-2. Cell. 2022

Chapter 4

COVID-19 Response in Uzbekistan: From RT-PCR Test System to the Clinical Trial of Subunit Vaccine

Shahlo Turdikulova, Dilbar Dalimova, Alisher Abdullaev, Muzaffar Muminov, Wang Ruyue, Liu Pengfei, Erkin Musabaev, Bahodir Yusupaliev, Botir Kurbanov and Ibrokhim Y. Abdurakhmonov

Abstract

The coronavirus pandemic showed the need for urgently improvement of different sectors in Uzbekistan, especially, the healthcare system and the biopharma industries. Uzbekistan government and private sectors have taken comprehensive measures to control the spread of infection in the country and tried to mitigate the impact of the pandemic. In this chapter, we discussed the primary measures taken to combat the coronavirus pandemic and the details of developing a local reverse transcription real-time PCR (RT-qPCR) detection kit as well as the experience of conducting the phase III clinical trials of the recombinant Uzbek-Chinese vaccine-ZF-UZ-Vac2001 against coronavirus infection. Finally, information is given on the mass vaccination campaign in the country, the difficulties encountered and the achievements made. The developed RT-qPCR detection kit was successfully implemented into production and have widely used for pathogen diagnosis. A total of 6965 volunteers over 18 years old participated in the clinical trials of ZF2001 and the vaccine had an efficacy level of 84.8%. More than 67.6 million doses were administered using seven types of anti-COVID vaccines in the country. The pandemics urged the country to establish a scientific and technical base that aimed at quickly responding to potential future challenges and emergencies.

Keywords: COVID-19, SARS-CoV-2, clinical trials, vaccination, vaccine, Uzbekistan

1. Introduction

The beginning of 2020 was alarming: the news of the impending coronavirus forced all countries to start preparing for the approaching infection. The wide spread of the COVID-19 pandemic has harmed the entire world showing the need for a more developed healthcare system to prevent such large-scale pandemics. A current advance in molecular diagnostic technology has enabled scientists to rapidly characterize the novel virus and deploy diagnostic tests [1]. The first months of the pandemic resulted not only in absence of approved therapeutics and vaccines but also in rapid diagnostic tests, especially in developing countries. To fill the lack of diagnostic tests, some low- and middle-income countries including Uzbekistan were forced to develop and launch their own diagnostic kits [2–4]. In addition to diagnostic kits, for early diagnosis of the disease, leading countries for R&D-driven biotech have developed several vaccines against COVID-19 at once. The rapidly growing infection rate of COVID-19 worldwide during 2020 stimulated international alliances and government efforts to urgently organize resources to make multiple vaccine types and conduct clinical trials on shortened timelines.

One of the first vaccines to successfully pass the third phase of clinical trials was BNT162b2 (Pfizer-BioNTech) a nucleoside-modified RNA encoding the SARS-CoV-2 full-length spike. A total of 43,548 participants underwent randomized controlled trials resulted in 95% of efficacy in preventing Covid-19 (95% credible interval, 90.3 to 97.6). Moreover, similar efficacy of BNT162b2 was observed across subgroups defined by age, sex, race, ethnicity, baseline body-mass index, and the presence of coexisting conditions [5]. This vaccine was widely used later against COVID-19. Another vaccine type, Ad26.COV2.S (Janssen; Johnson & Johnson) comprises a recombinant, replication-incompetent human adenovirus type 26 vector encoding a full-length, membrane-bound SARS-CoV-2 spike protein that was less efficient (66.9%; 95% CI 59.0 to 73.4) [6]. Subsequently, other vaccines successfully passed the 3-d phase of clinical trials worldwide, among them CoronaVac (Sinovac), an inactivated whole-virion SARS-CoV-2 vaccine yielding efficacy of 83.5% [7], mRNA-1273 (Moderna) a lipid nanoparticle-encapsulated mRNA-based vaccine that encodes full-length spike protein yielding efficacy of 94.1% [8].

Uzbekistan, along with many other countries, has suffered in many ways due to the COVID-19 pandemic, but the country has used methods based on world experience to combat the pandemic and mitigate its consequences. At the beginning of the pandemic, there was a great need for testing systems for the detection of coronavirus in Uzbekistan, as well as in many countries. Due to the global shortage of these test systems, it took a relatively long time to get test results. To overcome this problem, a project to develop a local qPCR diagnostic kit was initiated [9]. Currently, two local companies produce and offer RT-qPCR kits for the detection of genomic RNA [10, 11]. The scientists also determined the variants of the SARS-CoV-2 that are circulating in the territory of Uzbekistan using Next Generation Sequencing which helped to elucidate the distribution of SARS-CoV-2 variants in the country [12, 13]. For the first time, under the China-Uzbekistan partnership program, large-scale phase III clinical trials of the recombinant protein vaccine, ZF-UZ-VAC2001 were conducted in Uzbekistan to provide the population with a safe, highly efficacious vaccine as it is one of the priorities to control the disease [14].

Despite the fact that many measures have been taken to eliminate the coronavirus pandemic in our country, this pandemic showed that there is an urgent need for the development and production of national vaccines. Thus and because of the success in the development of local test systems, the government provided funding for research proposals on vaccine development from several scientific research institutes. The government also has initiated the construction of pilot and full-scale plants for the production of vaccines, which is not only critical to control the COVID-19 pandemic but also to increase our preparedness for the next possible emergencies [15].

2. Primary COVID-19 response in Uzbekistan

On January 29, 2020, a Special Republican Commission has formed to develop a program of measures to prevent the penetration and spread of coronavirus in the Republic of Uzbekistan [16]. In order to ensure epidemiological stability and protect public health, in the early stages of the pandemic, enhanced quarantine restrictions were imposed throughout the country. Pupils and students studied remotely. Air traffic and railroads were suspended. The work of sanitary and quarantine facilities was strengthened, and the regions' adapted quarantine zones were created. Our citizens from abroad were brought home on charter flights and placed in quarantine zones [17]. In Uzbekistan, since March 24, 2020, the wearing of medical masks had been mandatory, while in many countries of the world this issue had only just been discussed [18]. To provide sufficient masks to the whole 34 million population, the government decided to mobilize the textile enterprises to produce protective masks. For example, as the date of May 18, 2020, 275 businesses produced over 6 million masks and 45 thousand pieces of protective gowns per day [19].

Quarantine facilities for 20,000 beds were built in the Tashkent region, 7085 beds in Namangan, Samarkand, and Surkhandarya regions, and the Republic of Karakalpakstan, special hospitals for 4000 beds in the Zangiata district of the Tashkent region. Such special hospitals were also created in Nukus, Samarkand, Termes, and Pap districts [20, 21]. The state fully assumed the costs of fighting the infection, its detection, and treatment of citizens from coronavirus. A progressive package of economic measures was adopted to mitigate the impact of the crisis on relatively vulnerable sectors of the economy. An Anti-Crisis Fund had been created under the Ministry of Finance with an initial amount of 10 trillion UZS ($1 billion). Firms and entrepreneurs were provided with tax "holidays," a number of other benefits, and deferrals of loan payments. Social assistance had been organized for the most vulnerable groups of the population [22, 23].

At the expense of the allocated funds, it was possible to significantly strengthen the potential of healthcare: personal protective equipment, artificial lung ventilators, and other medical equipment were purchased in large quantities, including 878 thousand protective overalls, which allowed to maintain the health of medical personnel, avoiding mass infection of doctors as in some countries, the number of medical staff in clinics had fallen to a critically low level.

3. PCR test development

In the early beginning of 2020, there were only 15 PCR laboratories in the country in the Service for Sanitary and Epidemiological Welfare and Public Health, nowadays, there are 106 such laboratories, including 5 mobile ones [24]. In March 2020, the Special Commission instructed the Centre for Advanced Technologies under the Ministry of Innovative Development to develop and set up mass production of SARS-CoV-2 qPCR detection kits. During that period, a widespread lockdown was announced: all public and private institutions were closed, the movement of any type of transport was prohibited, and a regime of complete isolation of citizens was imposed. The R&D staff of the Centre involved in the project was mobilized to work in laboratories with permanent residence due to the lack of the ability to move around the city. The diagnostic kit "Biotest-SARS-CoV-2" for the detection of SARS-CoV-2 RNA by the real-time reverse transcription polymerase chain reaction was successfully developed in a very short time.

The kit is designed to specifically detect RdRp and N genes of SARS-CoV-2 in clinical specimens in accordance with protocols developed by Universitätsmedizin Berlin Institute of Virology (Charité, Germany) [25] and National Institute For Viral Disease Control and Prevention under the Chinese Center For Disease Control and Prevention (CCDC) [26].

Limit of detection (LoD) studies determined the lowest detectable viral concentration of SARS-CoV-2 (Genomic Copy Equivalents or GCE) that can be detected by the "Biotest-SARS-CoV-2" RT-PCR kit in a particular specimen type at least 95% of the time (95% of all true positive replicates test positive). The LoD was determined by serial dilution studies of the synthetic target gene of known concentration available from Molecular Cloud and produced by GeneScript [27]. For each concentration, qPCR was performed in four replicates per setup, the total number of setups was 3. The amplification was scored by threshold cycles (Ct) on a DT Light instrument (DNA Technology, Moscow, Russia) and Rotor-Gene Q (Qiagen, Hilden, Germany) according to the instructions for the kit.

The highest and the lowest concentration that was used in the reaction was 90,000 and 2 copies, respectively. According to experimental results, on DT Light instrument the detection rate of 2 copies in the reaction (or about 67 copies/ml) is 62.5%, whereas on the Rotor-Gene Q instrument the lowest detectable concentration is 5 copies per reaction. The LoD of viral RNA in a sample depends on the instrument, sampling, storage and extraction method, and dilution ratio. It was determined that the lowest concentration of viral RNA in a sample that can be detected on both Instruments (DT Light and Rotor-Gene) by the "Biotest-SARS-CoV-2" RT-PCR kit with the confidence of ≥95% is 10 copies per reaction or 330 copies per milliliter (0.33/μl). Thus, this concentration is the LoD that is detected in 100% of the tests.

The accuracy of coronavirus RNA detection using the "Biotest-SARS-CoV-2" RT-PCR kit was performed on clinical samples (37 positives and 45 negatives) in three independent laboratories of the Agency for Sanitary and Epidemiological Welfare of the Population (National analog of CDC) under the Ministry of Health of the Republic of Uzbekistan. The primers and probes included in the Biotest-SARS-CoV-2 real-time PCR kit were designed to detect specifically the SARS-CoV-2 coronavirus RNA genes based on the publicly available nucleotide sequences of its strains on NCBI and GISAID databases (https://www.ncbi.nlm.nih.gov/; https://www.gisaid.org/). Search through databases showed their 100% homology with all currently known strains of SARS-CoV-2. This was assessed with in silico sequence comparison analyses. Upon in silico analysis of the Biotest-SARS-CoV-2 real-time PCR kit, the assay design was found to detect all SARS-CoV-2 virus strains and it was found that the oligonucleotide design does not have homology and cross-activity with respect to other types of coronaviruses and non-SARS-CoV-2 species.

The Diagnostic kit was registered with the Agency for the Development of the Pharmaceutical Industry of the Ministry of Health (registration certificate No. № TB/IVI 00395/05/2CЮ dated May 7, 2020), and on May 9, an initial batch of 50,000 tests was released. On April 19, 2022, the intellectual property right for the diagnostic kit has been obtained (Patent # FAP02010). The first wave of COVID-19 in Uzbekistan had been started in July 2020, and lasted 3 months, at that time the production of qPCR kits reached 1 million per month and covered the needs of most state laboratories. In the context of a total shortage and the rising cost of diagnostic kits worldwide, only effective measures made possible to satisfy the need of Uzbekistan for COVID-19 diagnostic kits and overcome challenges with no bulk import. Currently, two companies are already producing COVID-19 diagnostic kits in the country [11].

4. Vaccine clinical trials, vaccination, and local vaccines

The next important step in the global fight against the pandemic was vaccine development and mass vaccination. As part of a partnership between the Ministry of Innovative Development and the Chinese Academy of Sciences, in July 2020, the question was raised about the need to create a vaccine and its further use. The Centre for Advanced Technologies under the Ministry of Innovative Development began cooperation with the Institute of Microbiology of the Chinese Academy of Sciences, and the pharmaceutical company Zhifei Longcom Biopharmaceutical Co. Ltd. on conducting phase III of clinical trials in Uzbekistan [28]. Noteworthy, none of the national medical institutions had previous experience in multicentre clinical trials for new drugs. Discussions involving scientists and leading doctors of the republic showed that there were doubts about conducting clinical trials at such a scale. Meanwhile, conducting the clinical trials would allow for analyzing the safety and efficacy of vaccines prior implementing to mass vaccination.

The vaccine formulated of protein subunit consisting of antigens with two SARS-CoV-2 spike RBD (HB-01 strain, residues 319–537, accession number: YP_009724390) connected in tandem (RBD-dimer), manufactured in the CHO ZN CHO K1 cell line. The advantages of this vaccine are included but are not limited to (1) the safety of this type of vaccine in comparison with other technologies and (2) storage conditions +4°C, which is important for Uzbekistan in terms of cold chain of storage and transportation [29]. A comprehensive study of the technology for obtaining a new vaccine, safety, and immunogenicity reports on phase I and phase II of trials made it possible to decide on our country's participation in clinical trials [30].

In October 2020, a tripartite memorandum was signed between the Ministry of Innovative Development, the Institute of Virology under the Ministry of Health of the Republic of Uzbekistan, and Zhifei Longcom Biopharmaceutical Co., Ltd. Thus, an agreement was reached to conduct the phase III of testing a vaccine against coronavirus in Uzbekistan. Prior to the start of clinical trials in Uzbekistan, the Pharmacological Committee of Uzbekistan conducted specification tests to analyze the effectiveness of antibody production and most importantly, evaluated the safety of the vaccine. In November, a group of Chinese researchers and specialists arrived in Tashkent. On our part, the Institute of Virology prepared a large group of doctors and nurses who were to work on the project that year, and more than 30 employees of the Centre for Advanced Technologies were allocated to the management and monitoring group. In total, more than a 100 medical workers were involved in the process, and later 36 more people were recruited to the Call Centre for daily monitoring of the health of volunteers.

At a meeting of the Ethical committee on December 10, 2020, an international, multicentre, double-blind, randomized, placebo-controlled III-phase clinical trial was approved in the Republic of Uzbekistan. The clinical trials were conducted according to the requirements of the international GCP standards and relevant regulations. Four vaccination sites were opened. Each volunteer was given a written consent form that contained the relevant details of the vaccine, the clinical trial, and the risks, and benefits associated with participation in the clinical trial. All volunteers were recruited based on voluntary principles after only signing a consent form and could suspend their participation at any time according to their will. To find eligibility the main health indicators were determined, and blood and swab samples were taken to determine previous COVID-19 and/or ongoing infection. Some of the subjects were not recruited for medical reasons, and others either had COVID-19 or refused to participate.

In Uzbekistan, between December 12, 2020, and Jun 30, 2021, a total of 13,855 volunteers underwent health screening, and 6965 people enrolled in clinical trials. Participants were stratified on the basis of age in two groups 18 ~ 59 years (6758 people) and ≥ 60 years (207 people) and randomly assigned into two groups to receive an investigational vaccine or placebo at a 1:1 ratio. A total of 6958 people (99.9%) were vaccinated with the first dose, 6717 people (96.4%) were vaccinated with the second dose, and 6395 people (91.8%) were vaccinated with the third dose. At least 7 days after the 3rd vaccination, a total of 53 COVID-19 cases were confirmed of which 46 were in the placebo group the vaccine showed an efficacy level of 84.8% (95% confidence interval, 66.2–94.2; **Table 1**).

Among the safety analysis set, 1301 (20.4%) participants reported at least one adverse event, with 709 (24.81%) participants in the vaccine group and 592 (23.36%) in the placebo group. Most of the reported adverse events 644 (20.22%) in the vaccine group and 517 (16.26%) in the placebo group were grade 1; 31 (0.86%) and 29 (0.83%), respectively, were grade 2; and 34 (1.07%) and 46 (1.44%) were grade 3 (**Table 1**).

During July–September, 2021 increase in COVID-19 incidence was observed in Tashkent with 84% of Delta strain detected by sequencing and PCR analysis. A total of 35 cases (1.08%) occurred among 3226 ZF-UZVAC-2001 group and 156 (4.84%) cases were confirmed in the 3221-placebo group. Vaccine efficacy for Uzbekistan trial group dropped from 84.8% to 80.2% (95% CI, 71.3–86.7). Other studies also reported a decrease in the effectiveness of the vaccine candidates against variants of concern including the Delta variant [31].

The research and organizational work of scientists from the Centre for Advanced Technologies and the Institute of Virology were highly appreciated by Chinese specialists and independent experts. The Chinese side announced the acceptance of Uzbekistan as a coauthor, and the vaccine was given the brand name ZF-UZ-VAC2001. Phase III of the research was carried out in five countries (China, Uzbekistan, Indonesia, Pakistan,

	Total cases	ZF2001	Placebo	Vaccine efficacy, % (95% CI)
Symptomatic COVID-19	53/6365 (0.8%)	7/3185 (0.2%)	46/3180 (1.4%)	84.8% (66.2 to 94.2)
Severe symptomatic COVID-19 and beyond	3/6365 (0.09%)	0/3185 (0%)	3/3180 (0.09%)	92.9% (52.4 to 99.8)
Death by COVID-19	0/6365 (0%)	0/3185 (0%)	0/3180 (<0.0%)	100% (−8.4 to 100)
Stratification by age				
Aged 18–59 years	52/6365 (0.8%)	7/3185 (0.2%)	45/3180 (1.4%)	81.2% (72.8 to 87.3)
Aged ≥60 years	1/207 (0.5%)			87.6% (2.5 to 99.7)
Adverse effects				
Total adverse effects	1301/6365	709/3185 (24.81%)	592/3180 (23.36%)	
Grade 1	1161/6365	644/3185 (20.22%)	517/3180 (16.26%)	
Grade 2	60/6365	31/3185 (0.86%)	29/3180 (0.83%)	
Grade 3	80/6365	34/3185 (1.07%)	46/3180 (1.44%)	

Table 1.
ZF2001 vaccine efficacy against COVID-19 with onset at least 7 days post-vaccination.

and Ecuador) with the involvement of 28,500 volunteers. The results of phase III clinical trial of the ZF-UZ-Vac2001 vaccine were published recently [32]. Vaccine efficacy after the third dose was 87.6% (95% CI, 70.6 to 95.7) in preventing moderate to severe forms of COVID-19. In total, out of 28,500 volunteers, 14,249 received the vaccine and 14,251 received a placebo, 647 of the volunteers were diagnosed with coronavirus, 221 of them—7 days after the third dose of the vaccine, 35 of those infected received the vaccine, and 186—placebo. These results demonstrate vaccine efficacy of 81.76% [32].

On March 1, 2021, the ZF-UZ-VAC2001 vaccine was registered with the Pharmaceutical Industry Development Agency of the Ministry of Health and approved for mass use in Uzbekistan. Thus, Uzbekistan became the first country in the world to approve and begin the mass use of a recombinant protein vaccine against coronavirus. On March 15, the vaccine was approved for use in China [33]. In April 2021, a mass vaccination campaign for adults over 65 and people at risk began, and a month later, vaccination of all populations was initiated [34]. All vaccination costs were made free for the population. The purchase of vaccines and the costs related to the vaccination program was covered by the state budget [35, 36]. To increase the vaccination coverage of the population, extensive explanatory work was conducted on the importance of vaccination and how they work. In addition, the introduction of various benefits to vaccinated people significantly increased the coverage of vaccination [37]. As the date of September 15, 2022, seven types of 44.2 million doses of vaccines were imported and 27.5 million doses of vaccines were produced in Uzbekistan from which 26.6 million doses of ZF-UZ-VAC2001 and 881.8 thousand doses of two-component Sputnik V vaccine.

Up to date, 71.9 million doses of vaccines have been used of which the majority share (48.2 million doses) of the vaccines belonged to of ZF-UZ-VAC2001 vaccine. In addition to the protein vaccine, the following vaccines were used in the country: Astra Zeneca 2.6 M doses (4%), (2%), Moderna 10.7 M doses (16%), Pfizer-BioNTech 6.8 M doses (9%), Sinovac 2.0 M doses (3%), and Sputnik-V and Light 1.645 M doses (2%) (**Figure 1**).

A total of 21.5 million of population was included in target group for the mass vaccination according to their age. No people under 18 were included for the national vaccination program against coronavirus infection. A total of 21.1 million people received the first dose, 17.8 million received the second dose, and finally, 10.6 million

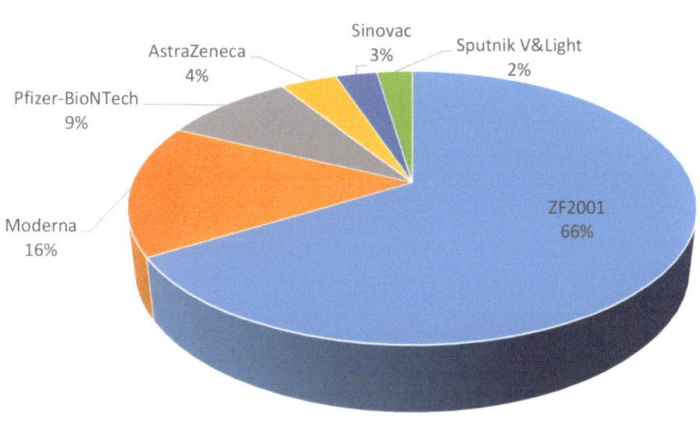

Figure 1.
The proportion of anti-COVID-19 vaccines used in Uzbekistan.

people received the third dose. From those 16.4 million people (76.6% of the target population) received a full vaccination course. Uzbekistan has become one of the countries where seven types of vaccines obtained using different technologies were simultaneously used. All vaccines showed good protection against severe forms of coronavirus: in persons who completed the full course of vaccination, there were practically no deaths, as well as no need for resuscitation [38].

In addition, scientists in Uzbekistan are conducting research on the development of vaccines against coronavirus. There are three vaccines listed by the WHO that are currently undergoing preclinical studies: the Renovac recombinant protein vaccine (developed by the Centre for Advanced Technologies), the Genovac DNA vaccine, and the Tomovac edible vaccine obtained by genetically modifying tomatoes (developed by the Centre of Genomics and bioinformatics, Academy of Sciences of Uzbekistan) [39].

5. Conclusions

The establishment of a special commission to fight against the coronavirus pandemic in Uzbekistan and the involvement of employees of state bodies with various backgrounds made it possible to consistently discuss the issues and make decisions in a short period. Multilateral cooperation in order to cover the need for vaccines became an important factor in the implementation of vaccination campaigns. The scientific and technical base created for the detection of the coronavirus also helped in the identification of new variants of the coronavirus. qPCR-based kits have already been developed that allow the detection of variants of concern such as Alpha, Delta, and Omicron. From a further perspective, the production of local kits for the detection of other important diseases may be implemented. In fact, there is already ongoing work to introduce new local test systems into the market. Uzbekistan's experience in conducting large-scale clinical trials stimulates local companies to conduct research on novel drugs. In addition, research teams are working on several vaccine platforms that may, in turn, enhance Uzbekistan's capacity for the development of national vaccines. Finally, these all initiatives including vaccine production capability can pave the way for increased resilience to combat infectious diseases and threats in the country.

Acknowledgements

We thank the governments of the Republic of Uzbekistan and the People's Republic of China for their invaluable support of scientific collaborations and for providing a fast-track approval process during the pandemic.

Conflict of interest

The authors declare no conflict of interest.

Author details

Shahlo Turdikulova[1*], Dilbar Dalimova[1], Alisher Abdullaev[1], Muzaffar Muminov[1], Wang Ruyue[2], Liu Pengfei[2], Erkin Musabaev[3], Bahodir Yusupaliev[4], Botir Kurbanov[4] and Ibrokhim Y. Abdurakhmonov[5]

1 Centre for Advanced Technologies under the Ministry of Innovative Development, Tashkent, Uzbekistan

2 Anhui Zhifeilongkoma Biopharmaceutical Co., Ltd., China

3 Virology Research Institute under the Ministry of Health, Tashkent, Uzbekistan

4 Agency for Sanitary and Epidemiological Welfare of the Population under the Ministry of Health, Tashkent, Uzbekistan

5 Centre of Genomics and Bioinformatics, Academy of Sciences of Uzbekistan, Tashkent, Uzbekistan

*Address all correspondence to: sh.turdikulova@mininnovation.uz; shahlo.ut@gmail.com

References

[1] Wu F, Zhao S, Yu B, Chen Y-M, Wang W, Song Z-G, et al. A new coronavirus associated with human respiratory disease in China. Nature. 2020;**579**:265-269. DOI: 10.1038/s41586-020-2008-3

[2] Munharo S, Nayupe S, Mbulaje P, Patel P, Banda C, Gacutno K, et al. Challenges of COVID-19 testing in low-middle income countries (LMICs): The case of Malawi. Journal of Laboratory and Precision Medicine. 2020;**5**:32 DOI: 10.21037/jlpm-20-84

[3] Fausto B, Nirmal G, Guiqiang W, Martin M, Luke O'N, Harald R, et al. Choice of SARS-CoV-2 diagnostic test: Challenges and key considerations for the future. Critical Reviews in Clinical Laboratory Sciences. 2022;**59**(7):445-459. DOI: 10.1080/10408363.2022.2045250

[4] VM C et al. Detection of 2019 novel coronavirus (2019-nCoV) by real-time RT-PCR. Euro Surveillance. 2020;**25**(3):2000045

[5] Polack FP, Thomas SJ, Kitchin N, Absalon J, et al. Safety and efficacy of the BNT162b2 mRNA Covid-19 vaccine. The New England Journal of Medicine. 2020;**383**:2603-2615. DOI: 10.1056/NEJMoa2034577

[6] Jerald S, Glenda G, An V, Vicky C, et al. Safety and efficacy of single-dose Ad26.COV2.S vaccine against Covid-19. The New England Journal of Medicine. 2021;**384**:2187-2201. DOI: 10.1056/NEJMoa2101544

[7] Mine T, Hamdi D, Murat A, et al. Efficacy and safety of an inactivated whole-virion SARS-CoV-2 vaccine (CoronaVac): Interim results of a double-blind, randomised, placebo-controlled, phase 3 trial in Turkey. The Lancet. 2021;**398**(10296):P213-P222. DOI: doi.org/10.1016/S0140-6736(21)01429-X

[8] Baden LR, El Sahly HM, et al. Efficacy and safety of the mRNA-1273 SARS-CoV-2 vaccine. The New England Journal of Medicine. 2021;**384**(5):403-416 DOI: 10.1056/ NEJMoa2035389

[9] A test system has been developed to detect the coronavirus in Uzbekistan. kun.uz [Internet]. 3 March 2020. Available from: https://kun.uz/uz/news/2020/03/24/ozbekistonda-koronavirusni-aniqlash-uchun-test-tizimi-ishlab-chiqildi [Accessed: 2022-08-15]

[10] The development of the test system created by our scientists has been further expanded. mininnovation.uz [Internet]. 27 July 2020. Available from: https://mininnovation.uz/news/2231#! [Accessed: 2022-08-15]

[11] PCR kit for the detection of RNA SARS-COV-2 "ROSSAmed COVID-19 RT-PCR" by RT-PCR in "real time". rossa.uz [Internet]. Available from: https://rossa.uz/en/covid-19-rt-pcr/ [Accessed: 2022-11-13]

[12] Ayubov MS, Buriev ZT, Mirzakhmedov MK, Yusupov AN, Usmanov DE, Shermatov SE, Ubaydullaeva KA, Abdurakhmonov IY. Profiling of the most reliable mutations from sequenced SARSCoV-2 genomes scattered in Uzbekistan. PLoS One. 2022;**17**(3):e0266417. Available from: https://doi.org/10.1371/journal.pone.0266417

[13] Abdullaev A, Abdurakhimov A, Mirakbarova Z, Ibragimova S, Tsoy V, Nuriddinov S, et al. Genome sequence diversity of SARS-CoV-2 obtained from

clinical samples in Uzbekistan. PLoS One. 2022;**17**(6):e0270314. Available from: https://doi.org/10.1371/journal.pone.0270314

[14] Vaccination statistics: Uzbekistan. 2022 [Internet] Available from: https://covidvax.live/location/uzb [Accessed: 2022-11-20]

[15] Decree of the President of the Republic of Uzbekistan, No. PP-4899 dated November 25, 2020. lex.uz [Internet]. 25 November 2020. Available from: https://lex.uz/ru/docs/5123684 [Accessed: 2022-11-20]

[16] Decree of the President of the Republic of Uzbekistan No. F-5537 dated January 29, 2020 [Internet]. 29 January 2020. Available from: https://lex.uz/docs/-4720398. [Accessed: 2022-11-20]

[17] Quarantine measures in Uzbekistan: Basic information. kun.uz [Internet]. 15 March 2020. Available from: https://kun.uz/uz/news/2020/03/15/ozbekiston-karantinda-asosiy-malumotlar [Accessed: 2022-08-15]

[18] Order of the Cabinet of Ministers of Uzbekistan: On additional measures against the spread of coronavirus infection. lex.uz [Internet]. 23 March 2020. Available from: https://lex.uz/docs/-4772484 [Accessed: 2022-08-15]

[19] Uzbekistan covered the population's need for masks. uzts.uz [Internet]. 18 May 2020. Available from: https://uzts.uz/ozbekiston-aholining-niqoblarga-bolgan-jehtiyozhini-qopladi/ [Accessed: 2022-08-15]

[20] Resolution of the Cabinet of Ministers of the Republic of Uzbekistan, No. 254 dated April 25, 2020. lex.uz [Internet]. 25 April 2020. Available from: https://lex.uz/docs/-4798481 [Accessed: 2022-08-15]

[21] Report: A special hospital built for coronavirus patients was opened in Zangiota district. kun.uz [Internet]. 5 July 2020. Available from: https://kun.uz/uz/news/2020/07/05/reportaj-zangiota-tumanida-koronavirus-bemorlari-uchun-qurilgan-maxsus-shifoxona-ochildi [Accessed: 2022-08-15]

[22] Decree of the President of the Republic of Uzbekistan No. PF-5969 of March 19, 2020. lex.uz [Internet]. 19 March 2020. Available from: https://lex.uz/docs/-4770761 [Accessed: 2022-11-20]

[23] The Government's report on the implementation of the state program was heard. senat.uz [Internet]. 5 February 2021. Available from: https://senat.uz/uz/lists/view/2371 [Accessed: 2022-11-20]

[24] Information on where to take a test for coronavirus was provided by region. review.uz [Internet]. 14 July 2020. Available from: https://review.uz/uz/post/koronavirusga-test-qaerda-topshirish-mumkinligi-togrisida-hududlar-boyicha-malumot-berildi [Accessed: 2022-11-20]

[25] Victor Corman, Tobias Bleicker, Sebastian Brünink, Christian Drosten, Olfert Landt, Marion Koopmans, Maria Zambon. Diagnostic detection of 2019-nCoV by real-time RT-PCR. who.int [Online]. 17 January 2020. Available from: https://www.who.int/docs/default-source/coronaviruse/protocol-v2-1.pdf

[26] Specific primers and probes for detection 2019 novel coronavirus. nmdc.cn [Internet]. 21 January 2020. Available from: https://nmdc.cn/nCov/en [Accessed: 2022-11-20]

[27] Plasmids for SARS-CoV-2 Research. molecularcloud.org [Internet]. Available from: https://www.molecularcloud.org/How-to-detect-the-2019-novel-coronavirus.html [Accessed: 2022-11-20]

[28] Uzbekistan poised to start trials on Chinese COVID-19 vaccine. euroasianet.org [Internet]. 10 December 2020. Available from: https://eurasianet.org/uzbekistan-poised-to-start-trials-on-chinese-covid-19-vaccine [Accessed: 2022-08-15]

[29] Dai L, Zheng T, Xu K, Han Y, Xu L, Huang E, et al. A universal design of betacoronavirus vaccines against COVID-19, MERS, and SARS. Cell. 2020 August 6;**182**(3):722-733.e11. DOI: 10.1016/j.cell.2020.06.035

[30] Yang S, Li Y, Dai L, Wang J, He P, Li C, et al. Safety and immunogenicity of a recombinant tandem-repeat dimeric RBD-based protein subunit vaccine (ZF2001) against COVID-19 in adults: Two randomised, double-blind, placebo-controlled, phase 1 and 2 trials. The Lancet Infectious Diseases. 2021 August 21;**8**:1107-1119. DOI: 10.1016/S1473-3099(21)00127-4

[31] Yan MZ, Yang M and Lai C-L. Review of Clinical Trials of COVID-19 Vaccination Booster in SARS-CoV-2 Variants Era: To Take It or Not To Take It. Frontiers in Drug Discovery. 2022;**2**:858006. DOI: 10.3389/fddsv.2022.858006

[32] Dai L, Gao L, Tao L, Hadinegoro SR, Erkin M, Ying Z, et al. Efficacy and safety of the RBD-dimer–based Covid-19 vaccine ZF2001 in adults. New England Journal of Medicine. 2022 June 2;**386**(22):2097. DOI: 10.1056/NEJMoa2202261

[33] New drug approvals: ZF2001, ZIFIVAX. newdrugapprovals.org [Internet]. 2021. Available from: https://newdrugapprovals.org/2021/06/20/zf2001-zifivax/ [Accessed: 2022-08-15]

[34] Mass vaccination against coronavirus kicks off in Uzbekistan. kun.uz [Internet]. 1 April 2021. Available from: https://kun.uz/en/news/2021/04/01/mass-vaccination-against-coronavirus-kicks-off-in-uzbekistan [Accessed: 2022-08-15]

[35] Who can take vaccines for free in Uzbekistan. review.uz [Internet]. 2 March 2021. Available from: https://review.uz/uz/post/kto-smojet-besplatno-vakcinirovatsya-ot-koronavirusa [Accessed: 2022-08-15]

[36] Resolution of the legislative chamber of the Oliy Majlis of the Republic of Uzbekistan, No. 763-IV dated February 22, 2021. lex.uz [Internet]. 22 February 2021. Available from: https://lex.uz/ru/docs/-5329280 [Accessed: 2022-11-20]

[37] Students who have been vaccinated against coronavirus will receive a 10% discount on the contract fee. gazeta.uz [Internet]. 4 July 2021. Available from: https://www.gazeta.uz/uz/2021/07/04/student-vacine/ [Accessed: 2022-11-20]

[38] The specialist explained that there will be cases of illness even after receiving the vaccine. kun.uz [Internet]. 27 June 2021. Available from: https://m.kun.uz/uz/news/2021/06/27/mutaxassis-vaksina-olgandan-keyin-ham-kasallanish-holatlari-bolishiga-izoh-berdi [Accessed: 2022-11-20]

[39] COVID-19 vaccine tracker and landscape. who.int [Internet]. Available from: https://www.who.int/publications/m/item/draft-landscape-of-covid-19-candidate-vaccines [Accessed: 2022-11-20]

Chapter 5

COVID-19 Response and Vaccination in Morocco: Efforts, Challenges, and Opportunities

Mohamed Khalis, Oumnia Bouaddi and Chakib Nejjari

Abstract

The Coronavirus pandemic has disrupted global health systems and has put enormous strain on fragile health systems worldwide. Despite the challenges that the Moroccan health system faces, the country's rapid and effective response to the COVID-19 pandemic has yielded positive results in terms of virus containment. A convergence of public policies has enabled Morocco to implement multifaceted interventions aimed at achieving large-scale vaccine coverage. These efforts have contributed to the success of Morocco's national vaccination campaign. While the immunization operation was not devoid of challenges, this experience has paved the way for Morocco to expand its disease surveillance system and explore its potential as a key actor in vaccine and bio-therapeutics supply on the continent.

Keywords: COVID-19, SARS-CoV-2, immunization, vaccine, infection prevention and control, pandemics, Morocco

1. Introduction

The COVID-19 pandemic and its spillover effects have disrupted global health systems around the world. Morocco has notoriously made major strides in the management and control of long-standing infectious diseases such as tuberculosis. However, the COVID-19 pandemic has inevitably put the Moroccan health system under strain and resulted in collateral social and economic repercussions. The pandemic response in Morocco was characterized by a remarkable convergence of public policies in order to alleviate the burden on those who were most affected by the negative impact of the crisis. Morocco was involved in vaccination efforts early on through participation in clinical trials. Given the fragility of the national health system linked to low bed capacity and a shortage in the healthcare workforce, the country has rapidly and effectively mobilized immense resources and engaged in organized efforts geared toward achieving population immunity. In this chapter, we give an overview of the COVID-19 vaccination experience in Morocco and also highlight the challenges that have emerged and discuss future opportunities and prospects.

IntechOpen

2. COVID-19 response in Morocco

Morocco issued a National Response and Surveillance plan against COVID-19 as early as January 27th 2020, and a steering committee was established by the Moroccan Ministry of Health (MoH) to oversee the health response [1]. The National Public Health Emergency Operations Center (CNOUSP), based at the Epidemiology and Disease Control Directorate (DELM), was charged with spearheading the monitoring of the epidemiological situation and the coordination of the technical aspect of the response. Additionally, the CNOUSP played a pivotal role in informing various stakeholders and partners, the media, and the public [1]. Field epidemiologists and rapid intervention teams were deployed in order to fulfill these roles. In addition to these tasks, the Regional Public Health Emergency Operations Centers (CROUSP) also organized training and information sessions for healthcare professionals both in public and private healthcare facilities [1, 2].

The first case of COVID-19 in Morocco was first recorded and confirmed on March 2nd, 2020. A 39-year-old man from Casablanca traveled to Brussels 15 days ago and then to Italy and returned to Morocco in late February. A swab was taken and the result confirmed SARS-CoV-2 as the causal agent. Contact tracing was performed, and 106 contact cases were identified and followed up [3].

Shortly after the first case was reported, decisive actions were taken by the Moroccan authorities to curtail the spread of the virus. Robust events were canceled such as the International Agricultural Exhibition (SIAM) and the international Crans Montana Forum in Dakhla. More stringent measures were put in place such as a nationwide school suspension by March 13th and the suspension of all international flights by March 15th. This was followed by more closures of mosques, restaurants, coffee shops, spas, gyms, and clubs and nationwide country lockdown. Non-pharmaceutical interventions (NPIs) such as mask wearing and disinfection were put in place and reinforced. On April 7th 2020, mask wearing was made mandatory in public places and at work [4]. Concurrently, industrial units were readjusted to increase local production capacity of masks—up to 5 million units a day—and a decree was enacted to regulate the price. A state of emergency was declared by the Ministry of Interior on March 20th, and a full-country lockdown was put in place. Citizens were allowed to move within their living space, and a special authorization was granted by local authorities to individuals working in vital sectors. Violations of the state of emergency became punishable by law per a novel decree Law 2.20.292, which was passed unanimously [5]. A nationwide survey of Moroccan households performed by the High Commission of Planning (HCP) between April and June 2020 showed an overall good compliance with some NPIs such as handwashing (87.3%) and wearing masks (78.3%). Other measures were less popular such as physical distancing (31.3%) and going out less (19.8%) [6]. These measures, namely those related to movement restrictions, proved to be effective in controlling the viral reproductive rate [7] but have naturally led to challenges experienced by Moroccans abroad awaiting repatriation and also resulted in financial hardships among Moroccan citizens, particularly those working in the informal sector. Fortunately, the economic consequences of the crises were anticipated through the creation of a COVID-19 special fund following the orders of King Mohammed VI; this fund initially contained 1 billion MAD and was later enriched thanks to contributions from banks, the National Security and Territorial Surveillance, telecommunication companies, MPs, and other senior officials. Additionally, stipends were issued to citizens working in the informal sector and who did not benefit from the state-funded insurance scheme Régime d'Assistance Médicale (RAMed). Notwithstanding, some decisions were met with criticism by the public such as the sudden decision to confine a few cities prior to the celebration of Eid El Adha in 2020. These decisions created panic among the public and led to overcrowded roads and an increased risk of creating infection clusters [2].

By June 2020, "Wiqaytna"—Arabic for "our protection"—was created by the Moroccan Ministry of Health (MoH) and its partners and made freely available to all Morocco citizens. The aim was to facilitate contact tracing and surveillance efforts [8]. In a similar effort, the Moroccan Ministry of Interior launched a hotline "Allo 300" to receive reports on suspected cases and provide information to citizens about COVID-19. As of June 2022, there are 1,170,427 confirmed cases and 16,080 deaths due to SARS-CoV-2. The evolution of daily confirmed cases of COVID-19 up to June 2022 is shown in **Figure 1**.

Regarding infrastructure and equipment, the COVID-19 response in Morocco was marked by an increase in hospital capacity through the establishment of field hospitals and the increase in the capacity of existing structures, including bed capacity for intensive care and resuscitation units. Thermal cameras and thermometers were made available at all entry points in order to maximize early detection of the virus. As changes in the case definition occurred, Morocco adjusted its surveillance strategy at all entry levels. Concurrently, local mass production of masks and hydroalcoholic gel took place alongside efforts to regulate prices. Additionally, Morocco considerably reinforced its laboratory capacity. At the beginning of the crisis in 2020, only three laboratories had a PCR platform, this number gradually increased reaching 30 laboratories with PCR testing capacity as of September 2021, among which six are mobile laboratories [2].

In accordance with the recommendations of its National Scientific, Technical and Advisory Committee, the MoH issued a standardized treatment regimen for COVID-19 patients, which included the use of hydroxychloroquine (HCQ)or chloroquine (CQ), combined with azithromycin (AZM) as first-line treatment [2]. The Moroccan Anti-Poison and Pharmacovigilance Centre subsequently received reports of medication errors related to the administration of AZM [9]. Following these alerts, the MoH

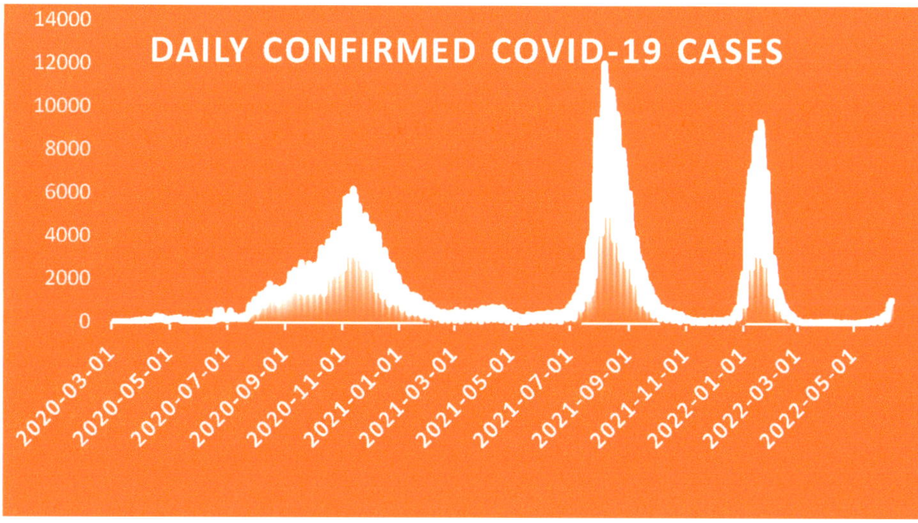

Figure 1.
Daily confirmed COVID-19 cases in Morocco.

issued recommendations directed at healthcare professionals and hospital directors in order to improve compliance with therapeutic guidelines [9]. In August 2021, the treatment regimen was updated to include Molnupiravir, an oral antiviral tablet recommended for non-severe SARS-Cov2 cases in high-risk individuals [10]. These updates were made in accordance with WHO treatment guidelines [11].

3. National vaccination campaign

3.1 Vaccination timeline, strategy, and efforts

Vaccinating the Moroccan population became a major public health priority, and remarkable efforts have been undertaken by the government to achieve large-scale immunization. In fact, preparations were arranged before the arrival of the first batches of vaccine doses into the country. Moroccan citizens and residents were notified about the procedure of setting up a vaccination appointment. The procedure simply entails providing one's ID card number to register and subsequently receive a place and date for their appointment. Any citizen or resident was automatically referred to the nearest vaccination center using its digitized identity card number. Concurrently, "Liqahona"—Arabic for "our protection"—the official portal of the COVID-19 vaccination campaign, was set up by the Moroccan MoH. This platform provides information about available vaccines, mechanisms of action, the vaccine development process and clinical trials, potential side effects, and enables individuals to verify their vaccination appointment [12]. Another channel by which Moroccan citizens could get informed about their appointment is simply by sending their identity card number to the toll-free number 1717. Upon receiving a second dose of the COVID-19 vaccine, individuals are able to download and print a copy of their vaccination certificate using the same platform. Similarly, an app named Yakadaliqah/Jawaz Asseha ("vaccine vigilance"/"Health passport" in Arabic) was made freely available in Google and Apple stores as well as a website version. The aim of this app is to allow citizens to benefit from remote monitoring by reporting any adverse event observed after the first and/or second dose of vaccine and enable continuous contact with the doctors at the local vaccination center [13]. These efforts were strengthened by mass communication campaigns through diverse channels such as national TV and social media. In fact, the MoH broadcasted SPOTS on national television channels such as SNRT, 2 M, and Medi1 in order to raise awareness, prevent pandemic fatigue, and encourage vaccination [2].

Morocco has participated in multicenter Phase III clinical trials of the COVID-19 vaccine Sinopharm in early August 2020 [14]. The trial was conducted at the Ibn Sina University Hospital and Mohammed V Military Training Hospital in Rabat and Ibn Rochd University Hospital in Casablanca [14]. The national campaign against COVID-19 kicked off in late January 2021. The campaign was completely free of charge to Moroccan citizens and foreigners residing in the country and was funded through the COVID-19 special fund. On January 22nd, Morocco received the first batch of the Oxford-manufactured AstraZeneca vaccine, consisting of 2,000,000 doses [15], and on January 27th, the first batch of the Sinopharm BIBP vaccine, consisting of 500,000 doses, arrived in the country. During this month, Morocco approved Sputnik V, Sinopharm BIBP, and Oxford-Astrazeneca and later on other vaccines were approved such as Sputnik V, Sinopharm BIBP, and Oxford-Astrazeneca, and later on other vaccines were approved such as Moderna and Pfizer-BioNTech [16]. Recognizing the critical role of cold chains in the success of immunization campaigns, the MoH worked closely with international organizations, foundations, and private sector partners, since the beginning of the national immunization campaign in January 2021, to expand and strengthen the country's cold chain capacity during the pandemic and beyond to also benefit the routine immunization program. In fact, four freezers were delivered to Morocco through the COVAX facility in 2021, which has increased storage capacity from 1.9 million to 4.1 million doses. Thanks to this facility, Morocco has received a total of 4,190,190 doses in 2021 [17]. The United States, COVAX's largest donor, has delivered 2,754,380 safe and effective COVID-19 vaccine doses including 2,449,980 Pfizer and 302,400 J&J doses [18]. The U.S. government has invested nearly $20 million in Morocco's COVID-19 pandemic response and U.S. military has invested over $3.8 million in field hospitals and laboratory assistance [19]. Furthermore, seven new ultralow-temperature freezers, funded by USAID and delivered through UNICEF Morocco, have allowed the country to double its storage capacity for COVID19 messenger RNA (mRNA) vaccines, including the Pfizer vaccine, which requires specific storage conditions at minus 80 degrees [17]. It is worthy of note that Morocco took part in the Chinese Sinopharm vaccine development process by participating in clinical trials. Therefore, it was among the first nations to receive the vaccine. In fact, 1 million doses of the Sinopharm vaccine were delivered to the country, which has allowed Morocco to scale up the vaccination campaign and target other subsets of its population. The vaccine roll-out in Morocco occurred progressively, and priority was given to those at high risk of contracting the virus and developing severe symptoms. The priority groups included health professionals aged 40 and over, public officials, the military, teaching staff aged 45 and over, as well as people aged 75 and older and individuals living with chronic diseases. Areas with high levels of circulating infection were also initially targeted [20].

Thanks to these joint efforts, as of June 8th, 2022, 24,839,199 of Moroccans have received their first dose of the COVID-19 vaccine, 23,321,341 have received a second shot, and 6,470,755 have received a third shot [21], thereby achieving the highest COVID-19 vaccination rate in Africa—63% of the total population are fully vaccinated [22]. This success has been attributed to the deployment of a smart vaccination campaign and technology, which has sped up the vaccine roll-out.

3.2 Challenges and opportunities

In discussing vaccination, the socio-behavioral aspect must not be omitted. The COVID-19 pandemic and the accompanied misinformation campaign led to the emergence of vaccine hesitancy among the world's population. Vaccine hesitancy presents a worldwide challenge that threatens to reverse years of progress made in infectious disease prevention and control. An initial survey conducted by the HCP after the first case was reported in the country, indicated that the acceptance rate was 68.6% among Moroccans [6]. However, the same report noted that nearly one household in 10 (11%) would refuse to get vaccinated [6]. More recent studies in Morocco reported low vaccine acceptance rates among health science students (26.9%) [23] and non-health-sciences students (35.3%) [24]. A similar study conducted among healthcare workers found a relatively high vaccination acceptance rate (62.0%). The main reasons of refusal or hesitation were concern about potential side effects (74.8%) and doubts about its effectiveness (47.8%) [25]. Similarly, one study was conducted among 3800 Moroccan citizens to evaluate the factors associated with COVID-19 vaccine acceptance using the Health Belief Model. The findings of this study were that perceived susceptibility and benefits were the strongest predictors of acceptance of the COVID-19 vaccine. Being female and having a chronic illness were also factors associated with a higher COVID-19 acceptance rate [26]. Throughout the pandemic response, the MoH deployed mass media campaigns to educate the public and promote vaccine uptake. Ultimately, legal action was taken against individuals who spread fake news about COVID-19 in order to prevent the undermining of public trust and prevent panic among the general public [27]. Examples of these legal actions were the arrests issued. Additionally, since the beginning of the pandemic, the MoH and the Ministry of Education urged citizens to fact-check pandemic-related information before sharing it. Furthermore, decision-makers in the country were the first to get the vaccine, which helped bolster public trust and dispel doubts surrounding the safety and efficacy of the vaccines. While vaccination is undeniably one of the most cost-effective interventions in the management of infectious diseases and to reduce the levels of circulating infection, compliance with NPIs and increased public awareness are of paramount importance in light of the emerging variants of concern (VoCs) and the waning efficacy of vaccines in the face of emerging variants.

The success achieved during the mass immunization operation compared with other countries in the region reveals the potential that Morocco holds in pioneering vaccine development and supply to the rest of the continent. In fact, efforts are already underway to accomplish this goal. In January 2022, Morocco has launched the construction of a vaccine manufacturing plant in the region of Benslimane, near Casablanca. This "fill and finish" site was launched in partnership with the Swedish firm Recipharm and was inaugurated during a ceremony attended by King Mohamed VI. This factory is expected to need an investment of almost $600 million and its objective is to achieve vaccine "self-sufficiency" for Morocco as well as to ensure coverage of 60% of the needs on the continent. This structure will allow for the transfer of aseptic filling and the manufacture of active substances of more than 20 vaccines among which are three COVID-19 vaccines [28]. It is worthy of note that Morocco is currently producing more than 3 million doses of the Sinopharm vaccine every month. This production is expected to reach 2O million doses by the end of the year. This was achieved thanks to the transfer of aseptic filling locally. While these prospects may be promising, the current crisis has not yet receded. In fact, the case count has been on the rise since the beginning of June 2022 as the country recorded a total of 1067 new confirmed COVID-19 cases as of June 12th [29]. This recent trend may force planners and decision-makers to reinstate movement restrictions, which may halt touristic activity—usually at its height during the summer season—and further delay the recovery of the Moroccan economy.

4. Conclusions

Morocco's strict and effective response to the COVID-19 pandemic has resulted in positive results in terms of preventing severe disease and limiting the spread of the virus. This experience has highlighted the country's potential in pioneering vaccine supply and promoting vaccine self-sufficiency on the continent. However, the harsh economic consequences, along with the emergence of other VoCs, may hinder these prospects. Therefore, careful planning needs to be undertaken to simultaneously address the collateral damage of the COVID-19 crisis, anticipate potential future threats, and explore current opportunities.

Conflict of interest

The authors declare no conflict of interest.

Author details

Mohamed Khalis*, Oumnia Bouaddi and Chakib Nejjari
International School of Public Health, Mohammed VI University of Health Sciences, Casablanca, Morocco

*Address all correspondence to: mkhalis@um6ss.ma

References

[1] Ministère de la Santé et de la Protection Sociale. Plan national de veille et de riposte à l'infection par le Coronavirus 2019 [Internet]. 2020 Jan [cited 2022 Aug 16]. Available from: https://www.sante.gov.ma/Documents/2020/coronavirus/Plan%20national%20de%20veille%20et%20de%20riposte%20à%20l%27infection%20par%20le%20Coronavirus%202019-nCoV.pdf

[2] Barkia A, Laamrani H, Belalia A, Benmamoun A, Khader Y. Morocco's National Response to the COVID-19 Pandemic: Public Health Challenges and Lessons Learned. 2021. Available from: https://pubmed.ncbi.nlm.nih.gov/34388104/

[3] Direction de l'Epidémiologie et de Lutte Contre les Maladies. Bulletin de l'Urgence de Santé Publique liée au COVID-19 CNOUSP, le 4 mars 2020 [Internet]. 2020 [cited: 2022 Jun 8]. Available from: https://www.sante.gov.ma/Publications/Bullten_pidmiologique/Bulletin%20de%20l%E2%80%99Urgence%20de%20Sant%C3%A9%20Publique%20li%C3%A9e%20au%20COVID-19%204%20mars%202020.pdf

[4] Organization for Economic Co-operation and Development (OECD). The COVID-19 Crisis in Morocco [Internet]. 2020 May [cited 2022 Aug 16]. Available from: https://www.oecd.org/mena/competitiveness/The-Covid-19-Crisis-in-Morocco.pdf

[5] Bulletin Officiel. Décret-loi n° 2-20-292 du 28 rejeb 1441 (23 mars 2020) édictant des dispositions particulières à l'état d'urgence sanitaire et les mesures de sa déclaration [Internet]. 2020. Available from: https://www.ilo.org/dyn/natlex/docs/ELECTRONIC/110337/137208/F-1115773749/MAR-110337.pdf

[6] Évolution des comportements des marocains face à la pandémie de covid-19 [Internet]. [cited: 2022 Jun 10]. Available from: https://www.hcp.ma/Evolution-des-comportements-des-marocains-face-a-la-pandemie-de-covid-19_a2572.html

[7] Ouchetto O, Drissi Bourhanbour A, Boumhamdi M. Effectiveness of containment measures to control the spread of COVID-19 in North Africa. Disaster Medicine and Public Health Preparedness. 2022;**16**(1):201

[8] el Otmani DZ, Sedrati H, Chaqsare S, Idrissi Azami A, Merzouki M, Raji M, et al. Moroccan digital health response to the COVID-19 crisis. Frontiers in Public Health. 2021;**13**(9):1105

[9] Ministère de la Santé. Centre Anti Poison et de Pharmacovigilance du Maroc [Internet]. [cited: 2022 Jul 25]. Available from: http://www.covidmaroc.ma/Documents/2020/coronavirus/corona%2003/Alerte%20sur%20les%20Erreurs%20Me%CC%81dicamenteuses%20lie%CC%81es%20a%CC%80%20l%E2%80%99administration%20de%20l%E2%80%99Azithromycine.pdf

[10] Covid-19. Mise à jour du protocole national thérapeutique (document) - Médias24 [Internet]. [cited: 2022 Jul 25]. Available from: https://medias24.com/2022/01/18/covid-19-mise-a-jour-du-protocole-national-therapeutique-document/

[11] WHO Updates its Treatment Guidelines to Include Molnupiravir [Internet]. [cited: 2022 Jul 25]. Available

from: https://www.who.int/news/item/03-03-2022-molnupiravir

[12] Campagne de vaccination contre le coronavirus au Maroc [Internet]. [cited: 2022 Jun 9]. Available from: https://liqahcorona.ma/fr

[13] jawaz asseha [Internet]. [cited: 2022 Jun 10]. Available from: https://jawaz-essaha.com/

[14] Ministère de la Santé et de la Protection Sociale. Stratégie nationale de vaccination contre le SARS-CoV-2 au Maroc [Internet]. 2021 [cited 2022 Aug 16]. Available from: https://www.wto.org/english/tratop_e/trips_e/11_presentation_bouchra_meddah.pdf

[15] Morocco gets 2 million AstraZeneca vaccine doses, first big shipment to Africa | Reuters [Internet]. [cited: 2022 Jun 9]. Available from: https://www.reuters.com/article/uk-health-coronavirus-morocco-idUSKBN29R1O0

[16] Morocco – COVID19 Vaccine Tracker [Internet]. [cited: 2022 Jun 9]. Available from: https://covid19.trackvaccines.org/country/morocco/

[17] Covid19 : Une campagne de vaccination réussie dépend aussi de la chaîne de froid | UNICEF [Internet]. [cited: 2022 Jun 8]. Available from: https://www.unicef.org/morocco/recits/covid19%E2%80%AF-une-campagne-de-vaccination-r%C3%A9ussie-d%C3%A9pend-aussi-de-la-cha%C3%AEne-de-froid

[18] Morocco – United States Department of State [Internet]. [cited: 2022 Jun 9]. Available from: https://www.state.gov/countries-areas/morocco/

[19] The United States delivers 850,590 doses of Pfizer vaccine to Morocco - U.S. Embassy & Consulates in Morocco [Internet]. [cited: 2022 Jun 9]. Available from: https://ma.usembassy.gov/the-united-states-delivers-850590-doses-of-pfizer-vaccine-to-morocco/

[20] Ministère de la Santé et de la Protection Sociale. Campagne Nationale de vaccination contre le virus de la COVID-19 [Internet]. 2021 [cited: 2022 Jun 13]. Available from: https://www.sante.gov.ma/pages/actualites.aspx?idactu=431

[21] Ministère de la Santé et de la Protection Sociale. Bulletin quotidien COVID-19 [Internet]. 2022 Jun [cited 2022 Aug 16]. Available from: http://www.covidmaroc.ma/Documents/BULLETIN/08_07_2022.Covidose.MAROC.pdf?fbclid=IwAR0UbY5SsaGV6zeK_V0sS24ARpUHEm8wbFfX1H_rqGdRO121qciLvgD6jLI

[22] Drissi Bourhanbour A, Ouchetto O. Morocco achieves the highest COVID-19 vaccine rates in Africa in the first phase: what are reasons for its success? Journal of Travel Medicine. 2021;**28**(4):1

[23] Khalis M, Boucham M, Luo A, Marfak A, Saad S, Aboubacar CM, et al. COVID-19 vaccination acceptance among Health Science Students in Morocco: A Cross-Sectional Study. Vaccines. 2021;**9**(12):1451

[24] Samouh Y, Sefrioui MR, Derfoufi S, Benmoussa A. Acceptance du vaccin anti-COVID-19 au Maroc: étude transversale auprès des étudiants. The Pan African Medical Journal. 2021;**2021**:38

[25] Khalis M, Hatim A, Elmouden L, Diakite M, Marfak A, Ait El Haj S, et al. Acceptability of COVID-19 vaccination among health care workers: a cross-sectional survey in Morocco. Human Vaccine Immunotherapy. 2022;**17**(12):5076

[26] Berni I, Menouni A, Filali Zegzouti Y, Kestemont MP, Godderis L, el Jaafari S. Factors associated with COVID-19 vaccine acceptance in Morocco: Applying the health belief model. Vaccines. 2022;**10**(5):784

[27] Morocco Continues Crackdown on Coronavirus Fake News [Internet]. [cited: 2022 Jun 11]. Available from: https://www.moroccoworldnews.com/2020/03/296591/morocco-continues-crackdown-on-coronavirus-fake-news

[28] HM the King Chairs Launching Ceremony of Covid-19, Other Vaccines Manufacturing Plant in Benslimane | Ministère de l'Industrie et du Commerce [Internet]. [cited: 2022 Jun 9]. Available from: https://www.mcinet.gov.ma/en/news/hm-king-chairs-launching-ceremony-covid-19-other-vaccines-manufacturing-plant-benslimane

[29] le Ministère de la Santé et de la Protection Sociale. Maladie due au nouveau coronavirus - La veille sanitaire au Maroc [Internet]. 2022 [cited: 2022 Jun 13]. Available from: http://www.covidmaroc.ma/Pages/Accueilfr.aspx

Section 3

COVID-19 Vaccines - New Directions

Chapter 6

The Silver Lining of the COVID-19 Pandemic: Fast-Tracked Vaccine Production and Approval

Wilson Lewis Mandala

Abstract

From the time when the smallpox vaccine was successfully produced in 1798, vaccines have proven to be the most reliable means for preventing and controlling most infectious diseases because they significantly reduce morbidity and mortality associated with life-threatening infectious diseases. During the pre-COVID-19 era, the development, testing, and final approval for vaccines would take as long as thirty years and this was regarded as a normal procedure by most regulatory bodies. However, the devastating COVID-19 pandemic witnessed the development and approval of several vaccines in just six months from when the first SARS-CoV-2 case was reported in Wuhan, China. The speed and apparent ease with which the COVID-19 vaccines have been produced and approved has introduced a paradigm shift in the vaccinology field, creating an environment within which the production of vaccines for most infectious disease now seems possible. This chapter delves into the vaccine production and approval process and discusses the benefits of vaccines, the types of vaccines, and how they work. It also explores how lessons from the COVID-19 pandemic can contribute toward the expedited development, trial, and approval of vaccines against other devastating diseases of equally high, if not higher, mortality rates such as HIV/AIDS, TB, and malaria.

Keywords: vaccines, COVID-19, HIV/AIDS, tuberculosis, malaria

1. Introduction

Over the years, vaccines have proven to be one of the most reliable means for preventing, controlling, and, in some cases, eliminating a number of infectious diseases. Where they have been used appropriately and administered at the right age and stage, both morbidity and mortality associated with the disease against which individuals have been vaccinated have been reduced or even eliminated [1]. Prior to the COVID-19 pandemic era, the development, testing, and ultimate approval of vaccines would take as many as 10 or even 30 years [2, 3]. However, the sudden advent of the COVID-19 pandemic witnessed the development of over a hundred vaccines against the viral disease (**Table 1**) some of which have already been approved (refer to Section 7.1) for use and have successfully saved millions of lives. More importantly,

	Vaccine platform	Number of vaccine candidates	% Total candidates
1	Protein subunit	43	34
2	Viral vector (non-replicating)	18	14
3	DNA	14	11
4	Inactivated virus	17	14
5	RNA	21	17
6	Viral vector (replicating)	2	2
7	Virus-like particle	5	4
8	rVV + APC	2	2
9	Live attenuated virus	2	2
10	nrVV + APC	1	1

Table 1.
Number (and percentage of the total) of different COVID-19 vaccines categorized based on the platform used to produce them (rVV = replicating viral vector, nrVV = non-replicating viral vector, APC = antigen-presenting cell).

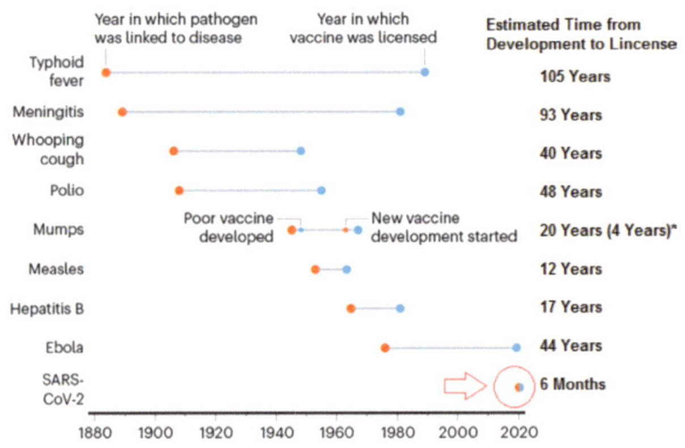

Figure 1.
Estimate duration (in years) from the time of establishing the causative link between a pathogen and the related disease to the time when a fully developed and tried vaccine is approved and licensed for use (adapted from Ball [4]).

the COVID-19 pandemic also experienced an astronomically expedited approval process for the new vaccines with some, such as the Pfizer COVID-19 vaccine, approved for use globally just after 6 months (**Figure 1**) from when the first SARS-CoV-2 case was officially detected and reported in Wuhan, China [3]. The speed at which these COVID-19 vaccines have been produced and approved has brought about a paradigm shift in the vaccinology world which some scientists and policymakers feel has completely revolutionized the vaccine development field. However, this watershed moment also raises some pertinent questions such as: are there any short-term and/or long-term effects on individuals who take such "seemingly" fast-tracked vaccines? Why have the vaccine-producing Pharmaceutical companies not been able to produce vaccines for other equally important and devastating infectious diseases such as HIV/AIDS, TB, and malaria in the past at an equally fast pace? Are there lessons or emerging innovative ways from the COVID-19 vaccine production platforms that could be used in an attempt to expedite the production of vaccines for these other infectious diseases that have been around for much longer than COVID-19? This chapter looks into the vaccine development world and highlights what can be adapted from the manner and speed at which the COVID-19-specific vaccines have been produced and approved.

2. History of vaccines

Vaccines are biological agents that can be used to safely induce an immune response against a specific antigen that is either derived from an infectious disease-causing pathogen or that is artificially manufactured [5]. Once the immune system is successfully and safely stimulated to respond to a vaccine, the vaccination process confers protection against infection or disease on subsequent exposure to that specific pathogen [5]. Edward Jenner is credited to have developed the very first vaccine in 1796–1798 using cowpox to inoculate humans against smallpox [6]. Prior to that, variolation, which was the ancient practice of inoculating human beings with biological material from an infectious disease-causing agent, was already in practice in various countries such as India, Turkey, and China centuries before Jenner's groundbreaking experiments [6].

Although Jenner's smallpox vaccine ended up being successfully used in various countries, the actual vaccination then was done from person to person with the biological material collected from one already vaccinated individual used to vaccinate others who were yet to be vaccinated [7]. The modern mode of vaccinating individuals was eventually developed by Louis Pasteur who developed vaccines by using agents extracted from disease-causing pathogens such that the effective vaccines against chicken cholera and human rabies in 1885 are accredited to him [7].

The next major innovation was the development of vaccines based on killed pathogens, which was done by two American scientists Daniel Elmer Salmon and Theobald Smith [6, 7]. This landmark was then followed by the vaccine development against typhoid, human cholera, and plague just before the end of the nineteenth century. Since then, many more vaccines have been developed as outlined in **Figure 2**.

During the twentieth century, vaccines against infectious diseases such as influenza and rotavirus were developed and these were either live attenuated, whole killed pathogens, or subunit vaccines that contained antigens such as protein, polysaccharides, or conjugated without the rest of the pathogen. In 1986, the first genetically engineered vaccine was developed and this was against Hepatitis B [7].

3. General composition of vaccines

The sole aim of vaccinating an otherwise healthy individual is to stimulate, pre-arm, and prepare the immune system in readiness for subsequent infections or diseases [5]. As such, the composition of each vaccine is essential as each primary ingredient is meant to be identified, recognized, responded to, and remembered by the highly developed and evolved human immune system during subsequent infections by the pathogen vaccinated against [7]. This being the case, the primary components of essentially all vaccines are protein antigens (with the exception of a few especially the polysaccharide vaccines) that are derived from the pathogenic organism that causes the infection one is being vaccinated against or synthetic antigens that

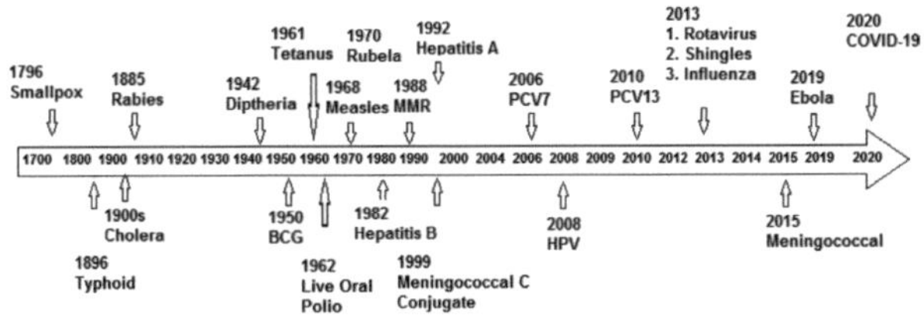

Figure 2.
Timeline for the development of various types of vaccines against different diseases.

resemble components of the pathogens that are manufactured [8]. In addition, vaccines would normally have natural or added adjuvants, which assist in boosting the immune response to the vaccine (immunogenicity).

Whereas the antigenic component of the vaccine directly induces the adaptive immune response toward a specific pathogen, in turn the adjuvants interact with the innate immune system through the pattern recognition receptors (PRRs) that recognize pathogen-associated molecular patterns (PAMPs) [9]. They would also contain stabilizers that maintain the stability and effectiveness of the vaccine after vaccine manufacture and during the storage period, some antibiotics aimed at preventing contamination during manufacturing stage, and emulsifiers such as polysorbate 80 and preservatives which protect any bacterial or fungal growth in the vaccine during the manufacturing and storage stages [8]. Various other products that are used during the vaccine manufacturing process sometimes end up as trace components of the vaccine and these include egg or yeast proteins, formaldehyde, and acidity regulators among other things [5].

4. How vaccines work

Vaccination, which is synonymous with vaccine administration, is the process whereby a biological product (natural or manufactured) from a known pathogenic organism is deliberately introduced into the body of an otherwise healthy human being with the aim of inducing the individual's immune response so as to confer protection against subsequent infections or disease caused by the specific pathogen [5, 8].

Once a vaccine is introduced into the body, its antigens are recognized by the host's antigen-presenting cells (APCs) such as dendritic cells (DCs), macrophages, Langerhans cells, and B cells. Antigen recognition is mediated in part by a set of proteins known as pathogen-associated molecular patterns (PAMPs) that are recognized by cognate proteins such toll-like receptors (TLRs) on the APCs' surfaces known as pattern recognition receptors (PRRs) [8]. While the antigen directs the specificity of the adaptive immune response against a specific pathogen, the adjuvants stimulate the innate immune response through the interaction of the PRRs and the PAMPs [9].

Once phagocytosed, internalized antigens are processed (digested) into peptide fragments and displayed on a major histocompatibility complex (MHC) either Class I (for CD8+ T cells) or Class II (for CD4+ T cells). Vaccine antigens that are produced in or enter the cytoplasm, such as live-attenuated viruses, are displayed on MHC Class I in a process known as the endogenous antigen-processing pathway. MHC-Class I-displayed antigens are recognized by the T cell receptors (TCRs) for CD8+ T cells.

In contrast, antigens that enter cells *via* a process of phagocytosis such as antigens introduced from killed or inactivated vaccines or recombinant proteins, or antigens that are secreted from infected cells, are displayed on MHC-II by the exogenous antigen processing pathway and are recognized by T-helper (CD4+) cells [5, 10].

The resulting activated APCs that are now presenting vaccine antigens on MHCs migrate to secondary lymphoid organs (SLOs) such as the draining lymph nodes, and spleen where they encounter naïve T cells in the T cell zones [11]. Interaction between antigen-presenting APCs and T cells through MHC/TCR binding leads to the differentiation and proliferation of naïve T cells into effector cells. In response to MHC-II/TCR binding, ligand-receptor interaction, and environmental support from cytokines, CD4+ T-helper (T_H) cells differentiate into T_H1, T_H2 T_H17, or Regulatory T cells. Of these, T_H1 cells secrete IFN-γ, which in turn stimulate the activation and expansion of cytotoxic T cells, whereas T_H2 predominantly secrete other cytokines such as IL-10, IL-4, IL-5, and IL-13 [5].

In contrast, following TCR/MHC-I interaction and help from T_H1 cells through INF-γ, CD8+ T cells differentiate into cytotoxic cells, which serve in part to recognize and eliminate infected cells thereby protecting the host against intracellular pathogens such as viruses. In addition to the effector cells that are generated in response to the presentation and recognition of vaccine antigens, both CD4+ and CD8+ cells also differentiate into memory cells such as central memory and effector memory among others. The memory cells are essential in responding and expanding the clonal pool upon antigen re-stimulation or subsequent encounter with the pathogen [12].

In addition to IFN-γ production, T_H1 cells are also involved in the production of IgG_1 and IgG_3 antibodies by different B cell subsets [5], whereas T_H2 cells secrete IL-4, IL-5, and IL-13, which promote the development, maturation, and differentiation of B cells into memory B cells (MBCs) and antibody-secreting plasma cells (PCs). The two other subsets of T cells, follicular T helper (T_FH) and T_H17, are essential for the generation of high-affinity antibodies and mucosal immunity, respectively. T_FH regulates B cell affinity maturation, selection of high-affinity germinal center (GC) B cells, and the duration of GC reaction [13, 14]. In turn, durable GC reaction favors the differentiation of GC B cells into high-affinity MBCs and antibody-secreting long-lived PCs (LLPCs) [5, 13].

MBCs are fundamental in vaccine-induced immunity since they can rapidly expand and differentiate into antibody-secreting plasma cells (ASPCs) upon re-encountering antigen thereby rapidly providing robust protection against disease-causing pathogen from where the antigen originated [5, 10]. LLPCs move from the draining lymph nodes (dLNs) germinal centers to the bone marrow to produce antibodies over a period ranging from few months to decades [12]. In addition, these LLPCs are terminally differentiated and, in contrast to MBCs, do not require reactivation or antigen re-encounter for them to produce antibodies. It is the high levels of neutralizing antibodies produced by LLPCs, which protects an individual against reinfection [5]. B cells, acting as APCs, are capable of recognizing and responding to vaccine antigen prior to engaging with T_H cells in what is known as T cell-dependent B cell activation. Just as is the case with the classical APCs, following vaccine administration, B cells recognize and internalize antigens and upon pattern recognition receptors (PRRs) activation differentiate into short-lived antibody-secreting cells, plasmablasts, that produce the first wave of antibodies. However, in the absence of help from T_H cells, B cells do not proceed to a stage of class switching into high-affinity antibody IgG secreting cells but instead will continue to secrete low-affinity IgM [8].

5. Types of vaccines

There are different ways of grouping vaccines depending on which characteristics are used. They can either be categorized as already licensed vaccines or those that are still being researched [8]. They can also be classified based on their ability to continue replicating once administered to the host such that some would be referred to as live vaccines and others as dead vaccines [5]. Vaccines can also be classified based on the technology platform utilized in producing them. Using this third criterion, vaccines can therefore be divided into the following types with some falling under the so-called Conventional Group and the others regarded as the so-called Next-Generation Vaccines (**Figure 3**) [8].

5.1 Conventional vaccine technologies

5.1.1 Live-attenuated vaccines

Live-attenuated vaccines, which are also known as replication-competent-attenuated vaccines, are prepared from weakened pathogens the virulence of which has been significantly reduced. The main feature of attenuated pathogens is that they characteristically mimic natural infection as they still maintain the intrinsic ability to infect host cells and replicate further within the host [15]. The main distinguishing feature of this type of vaccine is its ability to maintain the pathogen's replication potential without causing disease or attaining reversion to virulence.

Improved immunogenicity of live-attenuated vaccines is usually achieved through the activation of molecular sensors of the innate immune cells coupled with sustained antigen expression and presentation. Activation of pattern recognition receptors (PRRs) on classical antigen-presenting cells (APCs) such as dendritic cells (DCs) induces the upregulation of costimulatory molecules [16], and increases in the expression of various cytokines which, in turn, results in the differentiation and activation of the T_H1 cells thereby providing more potent cellular immune responses [10]. Most attenuated vaccines, like the one against smallpox which is now also being used in some countries against monkeypox, do not need an adjuvant and a single dose is sufficient to confer lifelong immunity [16]. However, the main disadvantage of these types of vaccines pertains to their potential to cause disease either in normal but most likely in immunocompromised individuals such as those infected with HIV. Although this type of vaccine is labor intensive in its production, they have been used successfully against such viral diseases as Polio and measles for decades (**Figure 3**).

5.1.2 Whole-inactivated (killed) vaccines

Although usually used interchangeably, the term "killed vaccines" is generally used in reference to vaccines for bacterial diseases, whereas "inactivated vaccines" relates to vaccines meant for viral infections [10]. These types of vaccines are derived from a killed form of virulent pathogens and typically stimulates a humoral-mediated immune response with the killing or inactivation process usually mediated by physical or chemical methods or a combination of the two.

These types of vaccines are comparably safer than the attenuated type since the inactivation or killing prevents any subsequent intra-host pathogen replication and potential gain of function mutations that could lead to reversion to virulence [8, 17].

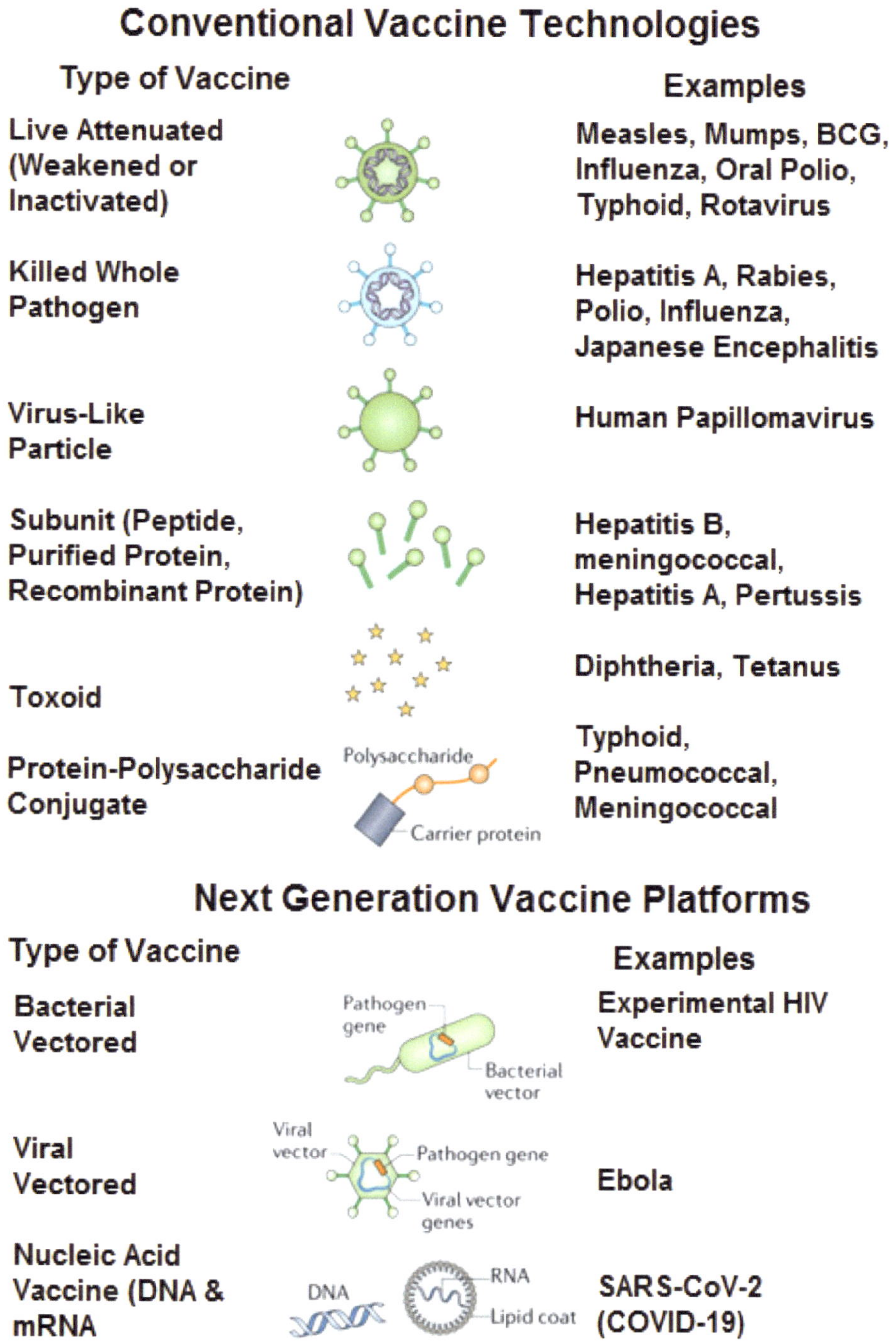

Figure 3.
Types of vaccines: a summary of different types of vaccines grouped based on the scientific technologies used for their manufacturing and indicating which pathogens they are currently being used against (adapted from Pollard and Bijker [5]).

In addition, these vaccines generate a much broad immune response against multiple targets since the whole pathogen is used during the immunization process. They are also less expensive to produce and because they are more thermostable, they can be stored for relatively long duration [7]. The main disadvantage of these types of vaccines is that they have limited ability to trigger cellular immune responses against intracellular pathogens. Furthermore, relatively large doses and regular booster injections are required for long-lasting protection due to lower immunogenicity. Although less expensive to produce, these higher doses and regular administration increase potential adverse events and manufacturing costs and reduce vaccine compliance. However, the efficacy of these vaccines can be substantially boosted by increasing the dose or the addition of an adjuvant in the formulation [10]. This type of vaccine has been used against diseases such as Hepatitis A, Zika virus, Poliovirus, Japanese Encephalitis virus, Diphtheria, and Tetanus [17].

5.1.3 Virus-like particles vaccines

Virus-like particles (VLPs) are macromolecular assemblies that are designed to mimic the morphology of a native virus in features such as size, shape, and surface proteins. VLPs can further be divided into two groups based on the presence or absence of a lipid envelope and the number of protein layers forming the capsid [18]. VLP-based vaccines are designed to target B cells and induce potent antibody responses following antigen presentation on MHC-II and activation of T_H1 cells. The process commences with VLPs being internalized by either classical or follicular dendritic cells or sub-capsular macrophages or B cells. The multivalent epitopes on the VLPs' surface are then displayed, which facilitate interaction with and crosslinking of B cell receptors (BCR).

Compared with other traditional vaccines, the high potency of this vaccine technology is associated with the multivalent interaction (increased avidity) with cells of the innate immune system, which results in their activation. In the past, this technology has been used to develop the human papillomavirus vaccine and is currently being used to develop vaccines against the Chikungunya, Zika [8], and SARS-CoV-2 viruses [19].

5.1.4 Synthetic peptide vaccines

Peptide-based synthetic vaccines, which are also known as epitope vaccines, are subunit vaccines which are manufactured from peptides. In turn, these peptides mimic the epitopes of the antigen that triggers direct or potent immune responses [20]. These peptide-based synthetic vaccines are relatively safer than live-attenuated or killed vaccines and have demonstrated efficacy against infectious diseases such as Hepatitis C, Influenza and recently COVID-19 [21]. In addition, the vaccines do not have any biological contamination since they are chemically synthesized and the peptides can be accurately designed for specificity. Furthermore, being synthetic, it is possible to design a single peptide vaccine that has multiple epitopes thereby generating immune responses for several diseases simultaneously. However, some of the main disadvantages of these types of vaccines include their poor immunogenicity and their instability once they are intracellular [20, 21].

5.1.5 Toxoid vaccines

Some pathogens, such as bacteria and not viruses, cause disease by secreting an exotoxin, which is responsible for the disease and not the pathogen itself. Examples of these pathogens include those responsible for causing diseases such as tetanus, diphtheria, botulism, cholera, and pseudomembranous colitis [10]. Toxoid vaccines, which are also known as fractional inactivated vaccines, are derived from the inactivation of such toxins and these vaccines generate an immune response against the disease-causing toxins. Inactivation of the toxin to convert it to a vaccine can be achieved by subjecting the toxins to chemicals such as formaldehyde, which results in altering either the structure of specific amino acids or in inducing minor conformational changes in the toxin structure. This in turn prevents and neutralizes any potential pathologic effects of the toxins on human tissues and also indirectly minimizes the invasiveness of the pathogen thereby rendering it harmless [22].

Since antitoxin responses typically do not target the actual bacterium, vaccine-mediated elimination of the disease-causing bacteria is not achieved. Instead, the bacteria are decolonized either through the normal immune response (with both the innate and adaptive arms involved) or through the use of appropriate antibiotics or *via* natural competition between the bacterial pathogen and the normal microbiota or a combination of any of these. Toxoid-specific T cell responses are mainly based on T_H1 cells [23], which then bridge the activation and differentiation of B cells into antibody-producing plasma cells and memory B cells that are essential during secondary infections. The addition of an adjuvant usually improves the efficacy and the longevity of the immune protection of this type of vaccine [23].

5.1.6 *Polysaccharide and polysaccharide conjugate vaccines*

When early bacteriological studies revealed that many pathogens were surrounded by a polysaccharide capsule and that specific antibodies against this capsule resulted in enhanced phagocytosis of the pathogen, the polysaccharide capsule was therefore considered a potential vaccine candidate [24]. Bacteria with a polysaccharide capsule include *Haemophilus influenzae*, *Neisseria meningitidis*, and *Streptococcus pneumoniae* and these cause infections such as meningitis, sepsis, and pneumonia, which are life-threatening [25]. Polysaccharide vaccines therefore are those that are derived from carbohydrate-based polymers such as peptidoglycans and glycoproteins that form the capsular structure of these pathogenic bacteria.

One drawback of this type of vaccine is that although they are extremely efficacious in adults generating high titers of serum antibodies, polysaccharide vaccines induce very low or have no immunogenicity in children aged less than 2 years [21]. This is the case because polysaccharides, unlike protein segments, are not processed and displayed on MHC molecules but remains T cell-independent [8]. The reason why only adults produce antibodies against these molecules is that a particular subtype of B cells, the marginal zone CD21 + B cells (MZB), which are found in the spleen, is critical in the detection and binding of naked or complement-coated polysaccharide antigens and this type of B cells is not found in infants below 2 years old [26].

This limitation of polysaccharide vaccines is overcome by adding adjuvants and forming glycoconjugates, which successfully results in inducing T cell response and improving their immunogenicity [8]. Polysaccharide conjugates are produced by covalent attachment of the polysaccharide with a carrier protein such as diphtheria or tetanus toxoids with the aim of boosting the vaccine immunogenicity and improving protection in infants and children [27]. With the polysaccharide chain conjugated to a protein, both of these molecules are presented on MHC Class II and this results in the recognition of the antigens by TCR and activation of the T_H response. The subsequent interaction between T_H cells and B cells improves titers and the quality of antibodies as well as B cell memory [27].

5.2 Next-generation (modern) vaccine technologies

Although the conventional vaccine platforms have proven to be so successful in the development of some extremely effective vaccines over the past decades, their production and testing process normally takes years (**Figure 1**). As such, using those classical platforms for developing vaccines against emerging pathogens that have pandemic potential such as SARS-CoV-2 is usually not feasible due to associated manufacturing limitations [28]. In light of this, there has always been a need to develop more modern platforms that could potentially be used to respond rapidly to pandemic threats. Such platforms also need to be versatile enough to be deployed in different parts of the world and can easily be scaled up for industrial production. This is where the so-called next-generation vaccine platforms perform better than the conventional ones. The following are some of these modern vaccine platforms.

5.2.1 Bacterial-vectored vaccines

Recently, genetically attenuated microorganisms, pathogenic, and commensal bacteria have been engineered to safely deliver recombinant heterologous antigens to stimulate the host immune system without causing any disease. The main characteristic of these live vectors is their capacity to stimulate humoral and/or cellular systemic immunity as well as mucosal immunity in some cases. As such, the use of this type of vaccines prevents pathogen colonization of mucosal tissues, which is the first point of contact for many infectious pathogens. In addition, delivery of DNA vaccines (refer to Section 5.2.3) and other immune system stimulatory molecules, such as cytokines, can be achieved using these special vectors, whose adjuvant properties and, sometimes, invasive capacities boost the immune response [28].

A good example is the use of live bacterial cells as carriers as one way of producing new vaccines [29]. Bacterial carriers can either be considered as non-pathogenic or pathogenic but attenuated carriers. Since most bacteria utilize the mucous membranes to gain entry into the human body for infection, using them as carriers makes it ideal for the administration of vaccines in the mucosal tissues thereby inducing mucosal immunity. However, one major disadvantage of this type of vaccines, especially when attenuated pathogenic bacteria are used, is the risk of infection, especially in children, the elderly, and immunocompromised individuals such as those infected with HIV. Therefore, non-pathogenic bacteria such as *Lactobacillus* species are considered to be better suited as vaccine vectors [30]. However, genetic engineering has made it possible to identify and delete specific genes responsible for bacterial virulence, which then allows for the attenuation of pathogenic bacteria such as *Yersinia pestis* to be used as vectors that cannot regain virulence [31]. Furthermore, as one way of improving antigen presentation for this type of vaccine, simultaneous expression and secretion of cytokines have been incorporated and this has improved the vaccine-induced immune response by both the innate and adaptive immune systems and also boosted immunological memory [32].

5.2.2 Viral vector-based vaccines

Viral vector-based vaccines are derived from viruses, which are genetically engineered to encode genes for one or several antigens cloned into the vector backbone. Viral vectors can either be engineered to be replication-deficient (replication incompetent), but still maintain their ability to infect cells and express the encoded antigen. On the other hand, replication-competent vectors are still capable of replicating and as such, they are considered to be similar to the classical live-attenuated vaccines [8].

This type of vaccine mimics natural infection to generate potent humoral and cellular (both T_H and T_C cells) responses [33]. In addition to being highly immunogenic, viral vector-based vaccines are easier to manufacture, and in some cases, safer in comparison with the inactivated, live-attenuated, and recombinant protein technologies. They are designed either for single administration or as a component of a mix-and-match heterologous vaccine regimen due to the strong immune response that they induce [34].

The main challenges with these vaccines include pre-existing immunity to the viral vector and reduced efficacy of subsequent administrations due to antivector immunity. In the case of SARS-CoV-2, vaccines were developed using vectors with low seroprevalence such as human adenovirus serotype 26 (Ad.26) used by Janssen/Johnson & Johnson and chimpanzee adenovirus (ChAd) vector used by Oxford/AstraZeneca. The vaccines were well tolerated and demonstrated an overall efficacy of 66% and 75% respectively in preventing symptomatic COVID-19 disease [35–38].

5.2.3 Synthetic DNA vaccines

DNA vaccines are relatively larger than mRNA, which tend to be polyanionic and sensitive to nucleases characterized by lower efficiency of passive entry into cells. Previous work has shown that synthetic DNA (SynDNA) that is delivered into the muscle is capable of transfecting different cell types including myocytes, keratinocytes, and tissue-resident APCs [39, 40]. Once it is internalized, DNA is translocated into the nucleus and transcribed into messenger RNA (mRNA), and the mRNA is then exported back into the nucleus for protein translation with the aid of ribosomes [21] and it is this nascent protein that serves as an antigen. Just as with exogenous antigen, this internally generated antigen can be presented on both MHC-I and II, which in part triggers a robust T cell response.

Tissue-resident APCs expressing the antigen of interest can move directly to the draining lymph node to initiate immune responses. In contrast, antigen expression on myocytes may generate immune responses by translation and secretion of the antigen into the local environment. This promotes the uptake and MHC class II-related cross-presentation by un-transfected APCs. B cells may also recognize secreted or shed protein, leading to their T cell-independent activation [40]. Irrespective of being secreted or shed, the soluble antigen can drain to lymph nodes, extending antigen presentation locally and in distal tissues, resulting in improved germinal center reactions and re-expansion of lymph-node primed CD4+ and CD8+ T cells. Transfected myocytes upregulate MHC-I and other co-stimulatory molecules such as CD80, and may contribute to T cell responses by priming naïve CD8+ T cells [41].

The fact that synDNA vaccines can induce both humoral and the cellular components of the immune responses is one special characteristic that improves their efficacy from that of the conventional vaccine technologies. Compared with the conventional inactivated, attenuated, and recombinant subunit vaccine platforms, synDNA vaccines are faster, cheaper, and easier to manufacture [42] and this makes this platform, as well as the mRNA one (Refer to Section 5.2.4), ideal for use in developing a vaccine in a pandemic setting. In addition, they can easily be lyophilized and are thermostable exhibiting much higher pharmaceutical stability than conventional inactivated or attenuated vaccines attributes that make them ideal for long-term storage under field conditions [8]. Although earlier studies raised some safety concerns with the persistence of synthetic DNA in the nucleus with an enhanced probability of integrating into genomic DNA (gDNA), recent experimental data suggest that this risk is extremely minimal. Despite positive clinical data, no DNA-based vaccine is licensed for human use as yet against any disease most likely because the generation of robust B and T cell responses requires at least a prime, and two or three boosters. However, about 14 DNA vaccine candidates for COVID-19 are currently under clinical trials (**Table 1**).

5.2.4 mRNA-based vaccines

The concept of mRNA-based therapeutics is not new since over three decades ago some researchers [43–45] successfully showed that mRNA extracted from cells and *in vitro* transcribed (IVT) mRNA could be delivered to cells and animals for protein expression. Despite encouraging results from subsequent studies, major limitations such as potent inflammation and reduced *in vivo* translation due to mRNA's short half-life were quickly recognized. Once these challenges were overcome, the platform improved enabling the successful development of mRNA vaccines and/or adjuvants, which elicited both antigen-specific cytotoxic T (Tc) cell and humoral responses [46].

mRNA vaccines can be divided into three major categories: conventional mRNA, self-amplifying mRNA (SAM), and circular RNA (circRNA). Conventional *in vitro* transcribed (IVT) mRNAs are relatively simple in their architecture and manufactured at a high yield using a cell-free template-directed enzymatic synthesis [47]. Depending upon the use of nucleoside modifications during manufacturing and synthesis, the conventional mRNA vaccine platform can be further divided into nucleoside-modified or non-modified mRNA. Nucleoside modifications have proven essential in successful clinical application of conventional mRNA vaccines. The significance of nucleoside modifications in ensuring the success of this platform was indicated by data for the COVID-19 vaccine from CureVac that showed disappointing results (47% protection compared to over 94% with the Pfizer/BioNTech and Moderna's vaccines). This significant difference in efficacy has been attributed to CureVac using unmodified mRNA, which has higher innate immunogenicity than nucleoside-modified mRNA [48].

As the name suggests, self-amplifying mRNA is engineered to include viral-derived molecular machinery such as alphavirus-derived replicases and conserved sequence elements (CSEs) to enable intracellular amplification of the mRNA sequence once it is administered [49]. The presence of replicase enzymes facilitates replication of the mRNA vaccine in the cytoplasm, resulting in efficient and long-lived transcription and protein expression. Since SAMs are relatively larger in size, their manufacturing is more complex and challenging compared with the conventional mRNA vaccines due to low yield, difficulty in purification, and susceptibility to autocatalysis and physical degradation. circRNA is a class of non-coding single-stranded RNAs generated through a non-canonical splicing event known as back-splicing in eukaryotic cells [50]. Some [51] have shown that circRNA generates potent antigen-specific CD4+ and CD8+ cellular and humoral immune responses in mice against SARS-CoV-2 and its emerging variants, therefore providing proof of concept for vaccine applications.

Immune responses to the mRNA vaccines are heavily dependent on the delivery system used [47], the immunogenicity of the encoded antigen, and the longevity and subcellular localization of antigen expression. This being the case, if these vaccines are delivered intramuscularly or intradermally, they tend to be highly immunogenic with the additional benefit of inducing local cytokine and chemokine production that initiates prompt recruitment of neutrophils, monocytes, and other cells to prime the immune responses. In contrast to synDNA, mRNA vaccines are directly translated into the cytoplasm, and the ensuing proteins are processed and presented in MHC class I and class II, followed by the presentation to CD8+ (T_C) cells and CD4+ (helper) T cells in the draining lymph nodes. Compared with DNA vaccines, the expression kinetics of mRNA vaccines is much faster, with the onset typically peaking 4 h after administration and this is the case because mRNA does not need to enter the nucleus. In comparison with viral and synDNA vaccine platforms, mRNA presents virtually no risk of integration into the genomic DNA, is more cost-effective, and is relatively easy to manufacture. That is what makes this platform so ideal for rapid vaccine production during a pandemic setting.

6. Vaccines production, testing, and approval process

6.1 Production

Different types of vaccines as highlighted in Section 5 are produced in different ways. However, the general outline of vaccine manufacturing generally comprises several basic steps that result in the finished product [52]. The first step is the generation of the antigen which is supposed to induce an immune response. This step includes the generation of the pathogen itself (for subsequent inactivation or isolation of a subunit) or the generation of a recombinant protein derived from the pathogen. In the case of viral vaccines, the viruses are grown in cells, which can be either primary cells, such as chicken fibroblasts (a good example is that of yellow fever vaccine), or continuous cell lines. In contrast, bacterial pathogens are grown in bioreactors using a medium developed to optimize the yield of the antigen while maintaining its integrity. Recombinant proteins can be manufactured in bacteria, yeast, or cell culture. The viral and bacterial seed cultures and the cell lines used for viral production are carefully controlled, stored, characterized, and, often, protected. The first step in manufacture is the establishment of a "master cell bank." From this bank, working cell banks are prepared that are used as the routine starting culture for production lots. The final vaccine is a direct function of its starting materials, and a change in this seed can be as complicated as initiating a new product development altogether [52].

The next step aims at releasing the antigen from the substrate and isolates it from the bulk of the environment used in its growth. This can be the isolation of free virus or of secreted proteins from cells or of cells containing the antigen from the spent medium and this is followed by the purification of the antigen [52]. For vaccines that are composed of recombinant proteins, antigen purification may involve many unit operations of column chromatography and ultrafiltration. For an inactivated viral vaccine, there may simply be the inactivation of viral isolate with no further purification. The formulation of the vaccine is designed to maximize its stability while delivering it in a format that allows efficient distribution. The formulated vaccine may include an adjuvant to enhance the immune response, stabilizers to prolong shelf life, and even preservatives to allow multidose vials to be delivered [53].

The formulation consists of combining all components that constitute the final vaccine and uniformly mixing them in a single vessel and this is done in a highly controlled environment to avoid contamination. During this phase, individual, thoroughly cleaned, depyrogenated, single-dose, or multidose containers are filled with vaccine and sealed with sterile stoppers or plungers. If the vaccine is to be lyophilized, the vial stoppers are only partially inserted so that moisture can escape during the lyophilization process, and the vials are moved to a lyophilization chamber. All vials receive outer caps over the stopper for container closure integrity [54]. In order to eliminate the introduction of extraneous viable and nonviable contamination, all filling operations are usually done in a highly controlled environment where people, equipment, and components are introduced into the critical area in a controlled manner. After filling, all containers are inspected using semiautomated or automated equipment designed to detect any minute cosmetic and physical defects. As with the formulation phase of the vaccine manufacturing operation, extensive control and monitoring of the environment and critical surfaces are conducted during operations. Quality control testing at this stage also consists of safety, potency, purity, sterility, and other assays that may be specific to the product. Storage at very low temperatures within the manufacturing supply chain may be used to reduce potency loss during storage [55].

6.2 Testing, approval and post-approval regulation

Vaccines are developed, tested, and regulated in a similar manner to other drugs based on stringent guidelines set by various regulatory bodies including the World Health Organization (WHO), the European Medicines Agency (EMA), and the United States Food and Drug Administration (USFDA) to name a few. However, in most cases vaccines are even more thoroughly tested than non-vaccine commodities firstly because the number of human subjects in vaccine clinical trials is usually greater and secondly because vaccines are normally administered to individuals who are not ill at the time of vaccination. The process of testing and approving new vaccines is generally divided into various stages but most regulatory agencies across the world usually divide it into preclinical (involving *in vitro* and *in vivo* testing in animals and generally exploratory in nature) and clinical (which involved clinical trials in human participants) stages (refer to **Figure 4**). However, regulation and oversight increase as the candidate vaccine gradually progresses through the process [57–61].

6.2.1 First stage: laboratory and animal studies

6.2.1.1 Exploratory stage

This stage involves basic laboratory research and often lasts 2–4 years (**Figure 4**). At this stage, scientists identify natural or synthetic antigens that could help prevent or treat a disease. These antigens may include virus-like particles, weakened viruses or bacteria, weakened bacterial toxins, or other substances derived from pathogens [58].

6.2.1.2 Preclinical stage

Preclinical studies use tissue-culture or cell-culture systems and animal testing to assess the safety of the candidate vaccine and its immunogenicity, or ability to provoke an immune response (**Figure 4**). Animal subjects may include mice and monkeys. These studies give researchers an idea of the cellular responses they might expect in humans. They may also suggest a safe starting dose for the next phase of research, as well as a safe method of administering the vaccine [58–60]. Researchers may adapt or modify the candidate vaccine during the preclinical state to try to make

DOI: http://dx.doi.org/10.5772/intechopen.107254

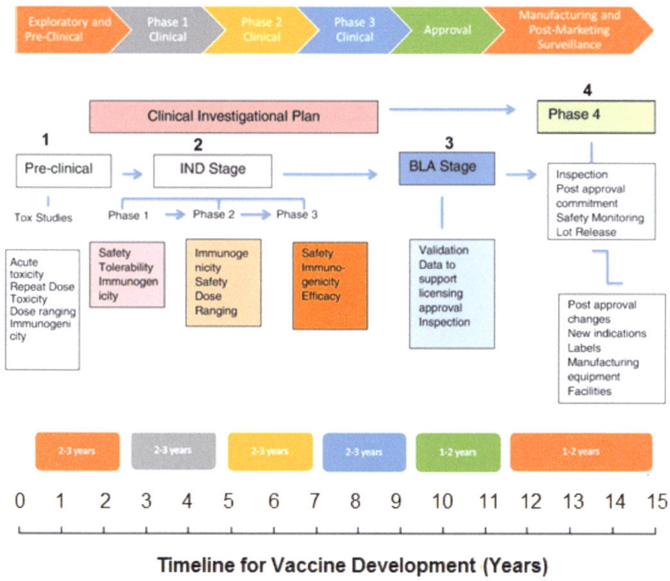

Figure 4.
An outline of the different stages testing, review and approval highlighting the preclinical, conducting of Phases I, II and III clinical trials, investigational new drug (IND) application stage, biologics license application and the phase 4 clinical trials that are usually conducted post-approval (adapted from Mao and Chao [56]).

it more effective. They may also do some challenge studies on the animals by vaccinating the animals and then infecting them with the target pathogen. Many candidate vaccines never progress beyond this stage, because they fail to produce the desired immune response. The preclinical stages often last 1–2 years and usually involve researchers in both private and public industries.

6.2.1.3 Investigational New Drug (IND) application

Under this stage, a sponsor, usually a private company, submits an application for an Investigational New Drug (IND) to a respective regulatory body such as the U.S. Food and Drug Administration. The sponsor describes the manufacturing and testing processes, summarizes the laboratory reports, and describes the proposed study. An institutional review board, representing an institution where the clinical trial will be conducted, must approve the clinical protocol [61]. Once the IND application has been approved, the vaccine is subject to three phases of testing.

6.2.2 Second stage: clinical studies with human subjects

6.2.2.1 Phase I vaccine trials

This first attempt to assess the candidate vaccine in humans involves a small group of adults, usually between 20 and 80 subjects. If the vaccine is intended for children, researchers will first test adults and then gradually step down the age of the test subjects until they reach their targeted age group. Phase I trials may be non-blinded (also known as open-label in that the researchers and perhaps subjects know whether a vaccine or placebo is used).

The main goals of Phase I testing are to assess the safety of the candidate vaccine and determine the type and extent of immune response that the vaccine provokes. In a small minority of Phase I vaccine trials, researchers may use the challenge model, attempting to infect participants with the pathogen after the experimental group has been vaccinated. The participants in these studies are carefully monitored, and conditions are carefully controlled. In some cases, an attenuated, or modified, version of the pathogen is used for the challenge. A promising Phase I trial vaccine candidate will progress to the next stage [58–60].

6.2.2.2 Phase II vaccine trials

A larger group of several hundred individuals participates in Phase II testing. Some individuals may belong to groups at risk of acquiring the disease. These trials are randomized and well controlled, and include a placebo group. The goals of Phase II testing are to study the candidate vaccine's safety, immunogenicity, proposed doses, schedule of immunizations, and method of delivery [58–60].

6.2.2.3 Phase III vaccine trials

Successful Phase II candidate vaccines move on to larger trials, involving thousands to tens of thousands of people. These Phase III tests are randomized and double-blind, and involve the experimental vaccine being tested against a placebo. One of Phase III's goals is to assess vaccine safety in a large group of people. Certain rare side effects might not surface in the smaller groups of subjects tested in earlier phases. A good example is that an adverse event related to a candidate vaccine could occur in 1 of every 10,000 people. To detect a significant difference for a low-frequency event, the trial would have to include 60,000 subjects, half of them in the placebo group [62].

Vaccine efficacy is also tested and the factors tested could include whether the candidate vaccine can prevent infection from the pathogen of interest and whether the infection leads to full-blown disease. More importantly, this stage also checks if the vaccine candidate leads to the production of antibodies or other types of protective immune responses related to the pathogen.

6.2.3 Third stage: approval and licensure

After a successful Phase III trial, the vaccine developer is expected to submit a Biologics License Application (BLA) to an appropriate regulatory body such as the USFDA, EMA, or WHO, which would then inspect the factory where the vaccine will be made and approve the labeling of the vaccine. After licensure, the regulatory body will continue to monitor the production of the vaccine, including inspecting facilities and reviewing the manufacturer's tests of lots of vaccines for potency, safety, and purity. The regulatory body has the right to conduct its own testing of manufacturers' vaccines [58–60].

6.2.4 Fourth stage: post-licensure monitoring of vaccines

A variety of systems monitor vaccines after they have been approved. They include Phase IV trials, the Vaccine Adverse Event Reporting System (VAERS), and the Vaccine Safety Datalink.

6.2.4.1 Phase IV trials

Phase IV trials are optional studies that drug companies may conduct after a vaccine is released. The manufacturer may continue to test the vaccine for safety, efficacy, and other potential uses.

6.2.4.2 VAERS

EMA (as well as individual EU member countries), USFDA and other regulatory bodies have established the Vaccine Adverse Event Reporting System (VAERS) with the aim of "detecting possible signals of adverse events associated with vaccines." A signal is regarded as evidence of a possible adverse event that emerges in the data collected being collected after a vaccine has been approved for us. Roughly, close to 30,000 events are reported each year to VAERS globally and as many as 15% of these reports describe serious medical events that lead to hospitalization, life-threatening illness, disability, or death [58–60].

VAERS is a voluntary reporting system such that anyone, including parents or friends of a patient or newly vaccinated individual or health care workers who suspects an association between a vaccination and an adverse event, may report that event and information about it to VAERS. The respective regulatory body then investigates the event and tries to find out whether the vaccination actually caused the adverse event.

7. COVID-19 vaccines: a game changer?

As mentioned earlier, the production of conventional vaccines is essentially based on reproducing the entire or part of the pathogen in some form either as an inactivated, live-but-attenuated, or as a subunit like a recombinant protein [63]. Although these modalities have worked successfully in the past against a number of pathogens such as measles and smallpox, they have had their own limitations. Over the years, advances in technology, immunology, vaccinology, structural biology of pathogens, and new vaccine platforms have contributed to the revolution in the vaccine development world. The success story of the COVID-19 pandemic has been greatly dependent on the earlier discovery that the virus' spike is the primary surface feature on coronavirus virions responsible for both attachment and entry into target cells [64].

Once the full sequence of SARS-CoV-2 was released, the race was on to develop a vaccine based on the virus's spike that could elicit the production of high titers of neutralizing antibodies efficaciously enough to control severe COVID-19 disease, hospitalization, and mortality. Currently, over three hundred COVID-19 vaccine candidates are at different stages of development and being tried (**Table 1**) with the following having already been approved for use by different regulatory bodies; the Pfizer-BioNTech BNT162b2 mRNA vaccine that has a reported efficacy of 95% [65, 66], the Moderna-US National Institutes of Health (NIH) mRNA-1273 vaccine with an efficacy of 94% [66, 67], the AstraZeneca-Oxford ChAdOx1 nCov-19 vaccine that originally had an efficacy of 67% [68], the Gamaleya GamCovidVac [Sputnik V] vaccine with a 91% efficacy [69], and the Johnson & Johnson [J&J] Ad26 COV2.S vaccine with 67% efficacy [66].

7.1 Types of COVID-19 vaccines and related platforms used

As of June 2022, a total of 320 vaccine candidates were in clinical (125) and preclinical (195) development stages globally with different developers using different platforms to manufacture their COVID-19 vaccines (**Table 1**). Based on history (refer to **Figure 1**), the fastest any vaccine had been developed in the past from pathogen sampling and identification to vaccine approval was the vaccine against mumps which took 4 years [4, 70]. However, for SARS-CoV-2, which was initially reported in Wuhan China in November 2019, by December 2, 2020, a period of less than a year (**Figure 1**), the Pfizer-BioNTech BNT162b2 mRNA vaccine with reported efficacy of 95% became the first fully-tested immunization to be approved for emergency use [65]. Within days, a few more vaccines were approved for emergency use. A number of factors have contributed to the speed at which these vaccines have been developed, fast-tracked through clinical trials, and approved for use.

One of the reasons for the rapid vaccine production was the knowledge and expertise gained through research conducted over the past years in vaccine production technology, which has largely benefitted from the advances in viral immunology, pathogen structural biology, and the availability of novel vaccine platforms listed in **Table 1**. For years, researchers had been working on related coronaviruses like the one that causes severe acute respiratory syndrome (SARS) and the ones responsible for the Middle East respiratory syndrome (MERS). Such work had enable the researchers to gain vast amounts of knowledge on the viruses' structure, which in turn provided a basis for the development of possible vaccine candidates using various vaccine platforms. As such, by the time COVID-19 was finally declared to be a global pandemic by the World Health Organization (WHO) on March 11, 2020, biomedical and pharmaceutical research and development companies in the USA alone had well over 70 potential SARS-CoV-2 vaccine candidates and vaccine technologies [3].

Funding is the main factor that facilitates and supports all this work. It is well known that the slowest component of the vaccine development process is not actually finding the promising vaccine candidates but testing such candidates, which usually takes years. However, it is not just the availability of funds alone that is fundamental, how such funds are used and the prioritized activities being funded are just as important. Such tests would normally start with trying the vaccine candidates in animals before shifting to the three-phase clinical trials in humans and all this requires huge amounts of money. The billions of dollars that were promptly made available by world governments and international organizations made it possible for most pharmaceutical companies to expedite the process in some cases, as was the case with Pfizer/BioNTech, conducting their Phase 3 efficacy trials in 150 sites in USA, Argentina, Brazil, South Africa, Germany, and Turkey [65].

The third factor is somehow linked to funding but is mainly based on the global response to previous epidemics such as Ebola. Some have argued that most wealthy countries, pharmaceutical companies, and international organizations only made the billion-dollars funding available to combat COVID-19 when they realized that their own economies were at risk of being severely devastated if the pandemic could be protracted [4]. This argument is supported by the observed country-based development of COVID-19 vaccines, which included the work of Sinovac and Sinopharm groups in China, India's Covaxin from Bharat Biotech, and the Russian Gamaleya rAd vaccine [3]. This observation, therefore, could be one of the main reasons why vaccine development for diseases such as malaria, TB, and HIV, which do not pose too much of a problem to wealthy country economies, may not be a priority for funding globally.

The fourth factor is the provision of a conducive environment for the development and approval of any promising vaccine candidates. The US government expedited the formation of public-private partnerships to safely and effectively accelerate the clinical development of the most promising vaccine candidates and also speedily put in place measures that could facilitate conducting of placebo-controlled efficacy and clinical trials of such vaccine candidates in line with the key endpoints and adherence to FDA protocols and guidelines [71, 72].

8. Current vaccine status for other diseases of interest

8.1 HIV/aids

Although the first cases of HIV/AIDS were detected in the USA in 1981, it took decades before any promising vaccine was even tried. Although HIV/AIDS has now been around for close to five decades, there have been no approved vaccines for the infection and the only HIV vaccine candidate, the RV144 which was investigated in the Thai clinical trial, has shown some promising results with an efficacy of 31% [73]. Although a number of mRNA vaccine candidates did show some promising results as an alternative to those produced through conventional methods, their further development and potential use have been restricted due to high intrinsic immunogenicity, easy degradation, and inefficacious *in vivo* delivery [74, 75].

Just as is the case with the various COVID-19 vaccines, an ideal HIV vaccine is expected to induce cell-mediated and humoral immunity. Antibodies that neutralize the virus would provide the first layer of defense, preventing infection of host cells upon virus entry into the body [65]. However, in the event that some virions succeed in evading the neutralizing antibodies, cytotoxic CD8+ T cells should then provide a secondary layer of defense, eliminating the earliest infected cells and preventing the establishment of a latent reservoir of HIV-infected. However, such a vaccine has so far proven to be elusive.

8.2 Malaria

A safe and protective antimalarial vaccine made up of irradiated *P. falciparum* sporozoites was first successfully administered to humans in the year 1973 [76], nearly five decades ago. Due to the complex life cycle of the parasite, three distinct vaccine development approaches that are currently being explored are based on the three distinct stages in the parasite life cycle essentially focusing on delivering antigen-specific vaccines as opposed to attenuated vaccines from live virus isolate [77].

8.2.1 Pre-erythrocytic vaccines candidates

These are designed to elicit a robust immune response that would prevent the sporozoites from invading and destroying infected hepatocytes [77, 78]. To date, the RTS,S/ has proven to be the most successful candidate among these vaccine candidates. The radiated circumsporozoite protein (CS) fused with a Hepatitis B surface antigen has been shown to be immunogenic conferring some protection, especially in children aged five or younger and subsequent trials in three African countries, including Malawi, have so far yielded very promising results [79, 80].

Although RTS,S has shown an efficacy of 55.8% in clinical trials in Africa [80], a new anti-malarial circumsporozoite protein-based vaccine, R21 with a Matrix-M™ (MM) adjuvant, has recently reported as high as 77% efficacy at high-dose adjuvant groups in preliminary clinical trials conducted in Burkina Faso [81]. If subsequent trials currently underway replicate such promising results, the introduction of the R21/MM vaccine could prove to be the turning point in the fight against malaria.

The recent success stories of mRNA-based vaccines against SARS-CoV-2 have prompted some investigators to explore if similar approaches could prove to be equally successful against malaria. A recent study [82] has shown some very promising results with an mRNA-based vaccine, which, similar to RTS,S, relies on *P. falciparum* circumsporozoite protein (PfCSP) to generate an immune response. However, unlike RTS,S, instead of administering a version of the protein directly, this vaccine introduces the mRNA specific for the PfCSP, which the instructs the cells to synthesize their own circumsporozoite protein that triggers a protective response against malaria [82]. Since this approach interrupts the malaria infection at a stage before the parasite reaches the RBCs, results in the mice models show that mRNA confers sterile protection against *P. bergheii* making it a very promising vaccine candidate for humans.

8.3 Erythrocytic vaccine candidates

These blood-stage vaccine candidates, including PfRH5, are designed to block the rapid invasion of RBCs by the parasites and their fast asexual reproduction once they are in RBCs. Since the blood stage is the stage when malaria-related symptoms manifest, with over 40,000 merozoites released for each infected hepatocyte, this is an important stage to disrupt. An ideal blood-stage vaccine should therefore aim to reduce the number of merozoites infecting RBCs rather than completely block their replication [80]. This being the case, currently there are no blood-stage vaccine candidates that have been as successful as the RTS,S vaccine.

8.4 Transmission blocking vaccine (TBV)

These vaccine candidates target the sexual reproduction stages in the mosquito gut to stop the parasite from spreading further. This is an indirect approach to a vaccine since the individual who gets vaccinated is not protected but rather prevents subsequent infections [79, 80]. The *Pfs*25-EPA vaccine candidate is designed on the basis that those vaccinated will produce specific antibodies against the specific antigen so that if a mosquito feeds on this person it will take up some of these antibodies into its stomach. Once they are in the mosquito's stomach, the antibodies will encounter the antigen, enabling them to interfere with the parasite's development and ultimately kill the parasite such that when the mosquito has its next blood meal it will not introduce any infectious parasites into the injected person [80].

8.5 Tuberculosis (TB)

8.5.1 BCG

Mycobacterium tuberculosis (Mtb) is associated with the highest annual mortality globally than any other infectious pathogen, but to date, there is only one licensed vaccine, Bacille Calmette Guerin (BCG) against the disease, and this vaccine has been in use for nearly hundred years. Unfortunately, BCG efficacy wanes in adolescents [83] and is known to offer little or no protection at all against adult-type pulmonary TB [84]. This being the case, despite universal infant BCG vaccination in all TB-endemic countries, close to 10 million people develop TB annually and of these, 1.6 million die from the infection [85]. As such, a more effective vaccine against TB is urgently needed.

8.5.2 mRNA TB vaccine

In 2004, a mRNA vaccine candidate that encodes the MPT83 antigen was reportedly successful in inducing protective cell-mediated and humoral immune responses against Mycobacterium Tb infection in mice models [86]. The protection was rather modest and was observed to be lower than that conferred by BCG and lasted for only 6 months. Unfortunately, this work has not been followed up since then probably due to the possible difficulties and costly process of developing the vaccine candidate.

8.5.3 DNA TB vaccine candidate

From 1996, well over 60 mycobacterial antigens have been identified as potential vaccine candidates. Subsequent immunization trials in mice using plasmid DNA encoding mycobacterial antigens have successfully triggered a robust T_H1 immune response characterized by high levels of IL-2 and IFN-γ [87]. The promising candidates include those based on cfp-10 antigen and ESAT-6 antigen. These vaccine candidates have the advantage that their use poses no risk of infection to the host, allows for antigen presentation to both MHC Class I and class II molecules, which could potentially trigger a much stronger and more robust immune response, are stable during storage, and can potentially elicit long-term immune responses [88]. However, since much of the work on these promising vaccine candidates has only been done on mice models, it is crucial that further research work should be done to determine their efficacy and graduate the most promising candidates to human clinical trials.

9. Conclusion

Vaccines still feature highly as the most effective means of reducing morbidity and mortality of most infectious diseases. In this COVID-19 pandemic era, they have once again proven to be the most reliable means of control against highly transmissible infectious diseases. The unexpected emergence of a previously unknown but highly contagious respiratory pathogen as the cause of a global pandemic has proven to be a blessing in disguise in terms of the global approach to vaccine development and approval. The speed at which these vaccines have been made available for use has been unprecedented and marks a watershed moment in the vaccinology world. However, the question still remains as to whether the same urgency with which COVID-19 vaccines were developed can be switched to the development of equally efficacious vaccines against other infectious diseases such as malaria, TB, and HIV, which have been around for much longer than COVID-19. One can understand why a vaccine for malaria, a disease caused by a protozoan, and for TB, a bacterial infection, might be harder to develop due to the more complex life cycles of the pathogens, but a vaccine against HIV, another viral infection, could be developed from some of recently tried and perfected vaccine platforms that have proven to be very successful in developing hundreds of effective vaccines against one viral disease. This is probably the best time to intensify the search for the most effective vaccines against these diseases although priority still seems to be focused on global preparedness for pathogen X in the future. The recent monkeypox outbreak, which has now been declared a "*global health emergency*" by the WHO [89], could serve as a justification for investing just as heavily in developing very effective vaccines against diseases that so far seem to be only prevalent in very few developing countries. The recent developments in the use of DNA and mRNA vaccines provide a great opportunity to fast-track the development and production of new and more efficacious vaccines for diseases that have been in existence for years such as TB and malaria. The recent establishment of the mRNA Vaccine Technology Transfer hub in South Africa [90] is a good example of how this technology can be fully utilized for new vaccine development and testing in countries where the diseases of interest are more prevalent and economically relevant thereby eliminating the recently observed vaccine equity during a pandemic setting [90, 91].

Acknowledgements

I would like to thank the Management of the Malawi University of Science and Technology for supporting my work.

Conflict of interest

The author declares no conflict of interest.

Notes/thanks/other declarations

None.

Author details

Wilson Lewis Mandala
Malawi University of Science and Technology, Thyolo, Malawi

*Address all correspondence to: wmandala@must.ac.mw

References

[1] Plotkin SA, Plotkin SL. The development of vaccines: How the past led to the future. Nature Reviews. Microbiology. 2011;**9**:889-893

[2] Han S. Clinical vaccine development. Clinical and Experimental Vaccine Research. 2015;**4**(1):46-53. DOI: 10.7774/cevr.2015.4.1.46

[3] Bok K, Sitar S, Graham BS, Mascola JR. Accelerated COVID-19 vaccine development: Milestones, lessons, and prospects. Immunity. 2021;**54**(8):1636-1651. DOI: 10.1016/j.immuni.2021.07.017

[4] Ball P. The lightning-fast quest for COVID vaccines—and what it means for other diseases. Nature. 2021;**589**(7840):16-18. DOI: 10.1038/d41586-020-03626-1

[5] Pollard AJ, Bijker EM. A guide to vaccinology: From basic principles to new developments. Nature Reviews. Immunology. 2021;**21**(2):83-100. DOI: 10.1038/s41577-020-00479-7

[6] Hsu JL. A brief history of vaccines: Smallpox to the present. South Dakota Medicine. 2013;**Spec no**:33-37

[7] Iwasaki A, Omer SB. Why and how vaccines work. Cell. 2020;**183**(2):290-295. DOI: 10.1016/j.cell.2020.09.040. PMID

[8] Ghattas M, Dwivedi G, Lavertu M, Alameh MG. Vaccine technologies and platforms for infectious diseases: Current progress, challenges, and opportunities. Vaccines (Basel). 2021;**9**(12):1490. DOI: 10.3390/vaccines9121490

[9] Medzhitov R, Janeway CA Jr. Innate immune recognition and control of adaptive immune responses. Seminars in Immunology. 1998;**10**(5):351-353. DOI: 10.1006/smim.1998.0136

[10] Baxter D. Active and passive immunity, vaccine types, excipients and licensing. Occupational Medicine (London). 2007;**57**(8):552-556. DOI: 10.1093/occmed/kqm110

[11] Chauveau A, Pirgova G, Cheng HW, De Martin A, Zhou FY, Wideman S, et al. Visualization of T cell migration in the spleen reveals a network of perivascular pathways that guide entry into T zones. Immunity. 2020;**52**(5):794-807.e7. DOI: 10.1016/j.immuni.2020.03.010

[12] Delves PJ, Roitt IM. The immune system. First of two parts. The New England Journal of Medicine. 2000;**343**(1):37-49. DOI: 10.1056/NEJM200007063430107

[13] Crotty S. T follicular helper cell biology: A decade of discovery and diseases. Immunity. 2019;**50**(5):1132-1148. DOI: 10.1016/j.immuni.2019.04.011

[14] Vinuesa CG, Linterman MA, Yu D, MacLennan IC. Follicular helper T cells. Annual Review of Immunology. 2016;**34**:335-368

[15] Mak TW, Saunders ME. 23—Vaccines and clinical immunization. In: Mak TW, Saunders ME, editors. The Immune Response. Burlington, MA, USA: Academic Press; 2006. pp. 695-749

[16] Pulendran B, Ahmed R. Immunological mechanisms of vaccination. Nature Immunology. 2011;**12**(6):509-517. DOI: 10.1038/ni.2039

[17] Sanders B, Koldijk M, Schuitemaker H. Inactivated viral

vaccines. Vaccine Analysis: Strategies, Principles, and Control. 2014;**28**:45-80

[18] Nooraei S, Bahrulolum H, Hoseini ZS, Katalani C, Hajizade A, Easton AJ, et al. Virus-like particles: Preparation, immunogenicity and their roles as nanovaccines and drug nanocarriers. Journal of Nanbiotechnology. 2021;**19**:59

[19] Xu R, Shi M, Li J, Song P, Li N. Construction of SARS-CoV-2 virus-like particles by mammalian expression system. Frontiers in Bioengineering and Biotechnology. 2020;**8**(862):1-6

[20] Bijker MS, Melief CJ, Offringa R, van der Burg SH. Design and development of synthetic peptide vaccines: Past, present and future. Expert Review of Vaccines. 2007;**6**(4):591-603. DOI: 10.1586/14760584.6.4.591

[21] Ada G. Overview of vaccines and vaccination. Molecular Biotechnology. 2005;**29**(3):255-272. DOI: 10.1385/MB:29:3:255

[22] Angsantikul P, Fang RH, Zhang L. Toxoid vaccination against bacterial infection using cell membrane-coated nanoparticles. Bioconjugate Chemistry. 2018;**29**(3):604-612. DOI: 10.1021/acs.bioconjchem.7b00692

[23] Mayer S, Laumer M, Mackensen A, Andreesen R, Krause SW. Analysis of the immune response against tetanus toxoid: Enumeration of specific T helper cells by the Elispot assay. Immunobiology. 2002;**205**:282-289

[24] Gotschlich EC, Irving G, Malcom A. Human immunity to the meningococcus: IV. Immunogenicity of Group A and Group C meningococcal polysaccharides in human volunteers. Journal of Experimental Medicine. 1969;**129**(6):1367-1384

[25] Lesinski GB, Westerink MA. Novel vaccine strategies to T-independent antigens. Journal of Microbiological Methods. 2001;**47**:135-149

[26] Kruetzmann S, Rosado MM, Weber H, Germing U, Tournilhac O, Peter HH, et al. Human immunoglobulin M memory B cells controlling Streptococcus pneumoniae infections are generated in the spleen. The Journal of Experimental Medicine. 2003;**197**:939-945

[27] Pichichero ME. Protein carriers of conjugate vaccines: Characteristics, development, and clinical trials. Human Vaccines & Immunotherapeutics. 2013;**9**:2505-2523

[28] Excler JL, Saville M, Berkley S, Kim JH. Vaccine development for emerging infectious diseases. Nature Medicine. 2021;**4**:591-600. DOI: 10.1038/s41591-021-01301-0

[29] Cardenas L, Clements JD. Oral immunization using live attenuated Salmonella spp. as carriers of foreign antigens. Clinical Microbiology Reviews. 1992;**5**:328-342

[30] Yurina V. Live bacterial vectors—A promising DNA vaccine delivery system. Medical Science. 2018;**6**(2):27-39

[31] da Silva AJ, Zangirolami TC, Novo-Mansur MT, Giordano Rde C, Martins EA. Live bacterial vaccine vectors: An overview. Brazilian Journal of Microbiology. 2014;**45**:1117-1129

[32] Chabalgoity JA, Baz A, Rial A, Grille S. The relevance of cytokines for development of protective immunity and rational design of vaccines. Cytokine & Growth Factor Reviews. 2007;**18**(1-2):195-207. DOI: 10.1016/j.cytogfr.2007.01.016

[33] Milicic A, Rollier CS, Tang CK, Longley R, Hill AVS, Reyes-Sandoval A. Adjuvanting a viral vectored vaccine against pre-erythrocytic malaria. Scientific Reports. 2017;**7**:7284

[34] Kunal S, Sakthivel P, Gupta N, Ish P. Mix and match COVID-19 vaccines: Potential benefit and perspective from India. Postgraduate Medical Journal. 2021;**98**(e2):e99-e101

[35] Folegatti PM, Ewer KJ, Aley PK, Angus B, Becker S, Belij-Rammerstorfer S, et al. Safety and immunogenicity of the ChAdOx1 nCoV-19 vaccine against SARS-CoV-2: A preliminary report of a phase 1/2, single-blind, randomised controlled trial. Lancet. 2020;**396**:467-478

[36] Feng L, Wang Q, Shan C, Yang C, Feng Y, Wu J, et al. An adenovirus-vectored COVID-19 vaccine confers protection from SARS-COV-2 challenge in rhesus macaques. Nature Communications. 2020;**11**:4207

[37] Zhu F-C, Li Y-H, Guan X-H, Hou L-H, Wang W-J, Li J-X, et al. Safety, tolerability, and immunogenicity of a recombinant adenovirus type-5 vectored COVID-19 vaccine: A dose-escalation, open-label, non-randomised, first-in-human trial. Lancet. 2020;**395**(10240):1845-1854. DOI: 10.1016/S0140-6736(20)31208-3

[38] Sanchez-Felipe L, Vercruysse T, Sharma S, Ma J, Lemmens V, Van Looveren D, et al. A single-dose live-attenuated YF17D-vectored SARS-CoV-2 vaccine candidate. Nature. 2021;**590**:320-325

[39] Marino M, Scuderi F, Provenzano C, Bartoccioni E. Skeletal muscle cells: From local inflammatory response to active immunity. Gene Therapy. 2011;**18**:109-116

[40] Hengge UR, Chan EF, Foster RA, Walker PS, Vogel JC. Cytokine gene expression in epidermis with biological effects following injection of naked DNA. Nature Genetics. 1995;**10**:161-166

[41] Shirota H, Petrenko L, Hong C, Klinman DM. Potential of transfected muscle cells to contribute to DNA vaccine immunogenicity. Journal of Immunology. 2007;**179**:329-336

[42] Tombácz I, Weissman D, Pardi N. Vaccination with messenger RNA: A promising alternative to DNA vaccination. Methods in Molecular Biology. 2021;**2197**:13-31

[43] Dimitriadis GJ. Translation of rabbit globin mRNA introduced by liposomes into mouse lymphocytes. Nature. 1978;**274**:923-924

[44] Malone RW, Felgner PL, Verma IM. Cationic liposome-mediated RNA transfection. Proceedings of the National Academy of Sciences of the United States of America. 1989;**86**:6077-6081

[45] Wolff JA, Malone RW, Williams P, Chong W, Acsadi G, Jani A, et al. Direct gene transfer into mouse muscle in vivo. Science. 1990;**247**(4949 Pt 1):1465-1468. DOI: 10.1126/science.1690918

[46] Conry RM, LoBuglio AF, Wright M, Sumerel L, Pike MJ, Johanning F, et al. Characterization of a messenger RNA polynucleotide vaccine vector. Cancer Research. 1995;**55**:1397-1400

[47] Alameh M-G, Weissman D, Pardi N. Messenger RNA-Based Vaccines Against Infectious Diseases. Berlin/Heidelberg, Germany: Springer; 2020. pp. 1-35

[48] Dolgin E. CureVac COVID vaccine let-down spotlights mRNA design challenges. Nature. 2021;**594**:483

[49] Magini D, Giovani C, Mangiavacchi S, Maccari S, Cecchi R, Ulmer JB, et al. Self-amplifying mRNA vaccines expressing multiple conserved influenza antigens confer protection against homologous and heterosubtypic viral challenge. PLoS One. 2016;**11**:e0161193

[50] Zhou W-Y, Cai Z-R, Liu J, Wang D-S, Ju H-Q, Xu R-H. Circular RNA: Metabolism, functions and interactions with proteins. Molecular Cancer. 2020;**19**:172

[51] Qu S, Yang X, Li X, Wang J, Gao Y, Shang R, et al. Circular RNA: A new star of noncoding RNAs. Cancer Letters. 2015;**365**:141-148

[52] Gomez, Robinson. Vaccine manufacturing. Plotkin's Vaccines. 2018;**51-60**:e1

[53] Rey-Jurado E, Tapia F, Muñoz-Durango N, Lay MK, Carreño LJ, Riedel CA, et al. Assessing the importance of domestic vaccine manufacturing centers: An overview of immunization programs, vaccine manufacture, and distribution. Frontiers in Immunology. 2018;**9**:26. DOI: 10.3389/fimmu.2018.00026

[54] Plotkin S, Robinson JM, Cunningham G, Iqbal R, Larsen S. The complexity and cost of vaccine manufacturing—An overview. Vaccine. 2017;**35**(33):4064-4071. DOI: 10.1016/j.vaccine.2017.06.003

[55] Gallo-Ramírez LE, Nikolay A, Genzel Y, Reichl U. Bioreactor concepts for cell culture-based viral vaccine production. Expert Review of Vaccines. 2015;**14**(9):1181-1195. DOI: 10.1586/14760584.2015.1067144

[56] Mao HH, Chao S. Advances in vaccines. Advances in Biochemical Engineering/Biotechnology. 2020;**171**:155-188. DOI: 10.1007/10_2019_107

[57] Singh K, Mehta S. The clinical development process for a novel preventive vaccine: An overview. Journal of Postgraduate Medicine. 2016;**62**(1):4-11. DOI: 10.4103/0022-3859.173187

[58] WHO Technical Report. Annex 1: WHO Guidelines on Clinical Evaluation of Vaccines: Regulatory Expectations. World Health Organization;WHO Technical Report. 2004;**924**:36-101. Available from: https://www.who.int/publications/m/item/guidelines-on-clinicalevaluation-of-vaccines-regulatoryexpectations. Accessed: September 12, 2022

[59] European Medicines Agency. Committee for Medicinal Products for Human Use. Guideline on Clinical Evaluation of New Vaccines (EMEA/CHMP/VWP/164653/2005). 2005. pp. 1-19

[60] U.S Department of Health and Human Services. Vaccine product approval process. U.S. Food and Drug Administration. 2018 [Accessed: July 22, 2022]

[61] U.S. Department of Health and Human Services. Investigational New Drug (IND) Application. U.S. Food and Drug Administration. 2017 [Accessed: July 22, 2022]

[62] Stratton K, Ford A, Rusch E, Clayton EW, editors. Committee to Review Adverse Effects of Vaccines; Institute of Medicine. Adverse Effects of Vaccines: Evidence and Causality. Washington (DC): National Academies Press (US); 2011

[63] Gerberding JL, Haynes BF. Vaccine innovations—Past and future. New England Journal of Medicine.

2021;**384**(5):393-396. DOI: 10.1056/NEJMp2029466

[64] Liu Y, Soh WT, Kishikawa JI, Hirose M, Nakayama EE, et al. An infectivity-enhancing site on the SARS-CoV-2 spike protein targeted by antibodies. Cell. 2021;**184**(13):3452-3466.e18. DOI: 10.1016/j.cell.2021.05.032

[65] Polack FP, Thomas SJ, Kitchin N, Absalon J, Gurtman A, Lockhart S, et al. Safety and efficacy of the BNT162b2 mRNA Covid-19 vaccine. The New England Journal of Medicine. 2020;**383**(27):2603-2615. DOI: 10.1056/NEJMoa2034577

[66] Pawlowski C, Lenehan P, Puranik A, Agarwal V, Venkatakrishnan AJ, Niesen MJM, et al. FDA-authorized mRNA COVID-19 vaccines are effective per real-world evidence synthesized across a multi-state health system. Med (N Y). 2021;**2**(8):979-992.e8. DOI: 10.1016/j.medj.2021.06.007

[67] Baden LR, El Sahly HM, Essink B, Kotloff K, Frey S, et al. Efficacy and safety of the mRNA-1273 SARS-CoV-2 vaccine. The New England Journal of Medicine. 2021;**384**(5):403-416. DOI: 10.1056/NEJMoa2035389

[68] Voysey M, Clemens SAC, Madhi SA, Weckx LY, Folegatti PM, Aley PK, et al. Safety and efficacy of the ChAdOx1 nCoV-19 vaccine (AZD1222) against SARS-CoV-2: An interim analysis of four randomised controlled trials in Brazil, South Africa, and the UK. Lancet. 2021;**397**(10269):99-111. DOI: 10.1016/S0140-6736(20)32661-1

[69] Logunov DY, Dolzhikova IV, Shcheblyakov DV, Tukhvatulin AI, Zubkova OV, et al. Safety and efficacy of an rAd26 and rAd5 vector-based heterologous prime-boost COVID-19 vaccine: An interim analysis of a randomised controlled phase 3 trial in Russia. Lancet. 2021;**397**(10275):671-681. DOI: 10.1016/S0140-6736(21)00234-8

[70] World Health Organisation. Mumps virus vaccines: WHO position paper. Weekly Epidemiological Record. 2007;**82**:49-60

[71] Fast-and-fit vaccines. Nature Biomedical Engineering. 2020;**4**(8):757-758. DOI: 10.1038/s41551-020-00605-9

[72] Corey L, Mascola JR, Fauci AS, Collins FS. A strategic approach to COVID-19 vaccine R&D. Science. 2020;**368**(6494):948-950. DOI: 10.1126/science.abc5312

[73] Rolland M, Gilbert P. Evaluating immune correlates in HIV type 1 vaccine efficacy trials: What RV144 may provide. AIDS Research and Human Retroviruses. 2012;**28**(4):400-404. DOI: 10.1089/aid.2011.0240

[74] Mu Z, Haynes BF, Cain DW. HIV mRNA vaccines-progress and future paths. Vaccines (Basel). 2021;**9**(2):134. DOI: 10.3390/vaccines9020134

[75] Khalid K, Padda J, Khedr A, Ismail D, Zubair U, Al-Ewaidat OA, et al. HIV and messenger RNA (mRNA) vaccine. Cureus. 2021;**13**(7):e16197. DOI: 10.7759/cureus.16197

[76] Clyde DF, Most H, McCarthy VC, Vanderberg JP. Immunization of man against sporozite-induced falciparum malaria. The American Journal of the Medical Sciences. 1973;**66**(3):169-177

[77] Tongren JE, Zavala F, Roos DS, Riley EM. Malaria vaccines: If at first you don't succeed. Trends in Parasitology. 2004;**20**(12):604-610

[78] Targett GA. Malaria vaccines 1985-2005: A full circle? Trends in Parasitology. 2005;**21**(11):499-503

[79] RTS,S malaria candidate vaccine reduces malaria by approximately one-third in African infants. malariavaccine.org. Malaria Vaccine Initiative Path. Accessed: [December 20, 2018]

[80] Vandoolaeghe P, Schuerman L. The RTS,S/AS01 malaria vaccine in children 5 to 17 months of age at first vaccination. Expert Review of Vaccines. 2016;**15**(12):1481-1493

[81] Datoo MS, Natama MH, Somé A, Traoré O, Rouamba T, Bellamy D, et al. Efficacy of a low-dose candidate malaria vaccine, R21 in adjuvant matrix-M, with seasonal administration to children in Burkina Faso: A randomised controlled trial. Lancet. 2021;**397**(10287):1809-1818

[82] Mallory KL, Taylor JA, Zou X, et al. Messenger RNA expressing PfCSP induces functional, protective immune responses against malaria in mice. npj Vaccines. 2021;**6**:84

[83] Sterne JA, Rodrigues LC, Guedes IN. Does the efficacy of BCG decline with time since vaccination? The International Journal of Tuberculosis and Lung Disease. 1998;**2**(3):200-207

[84] Mangtani P, Abubakar I, Ariti C, Beynon R, Pimpin L, Fine PE, et al. Protection by BCG vaccine against tuberculosis: A systematic review of randomized controlled trials. Clinical Infectious Diseases. 2014;**58**(4):470-480. DOI: 10.1093/cid/cit790

[85] World Health Organization. BCG vaccine: WHO position paper, February 2018—Recommendations. Vaccine. 2018;**36**(24):3408-3410. DOI: 10.1016/j.vaccine.2018.03.009

[86] Xue T, Stavropoulos E, Yang M, Ragno S, Vordermeier M, Chambers M, et al. RNA encoding the MPT83 antigen induces protective immune responses against mycobacterium tuberculosis infection. Infection and Immunity. 2004;**72**(11):6324-6329. DOI: 10.1128/IAI.72.11.6324-6329.2004

[87] Kaufmann SH, Hussey G, Lambert PH. New vaccines for tuberculosis. Lancet. 2010;**375**(9731):2110-2119. DOI: 10.1016/S0140-6736(10)60393-5

[88] Kim WS, Kim H, Kwon KW, Cho SN, Shin SJ. Immunogenicity and vaccine potential of InsB, an ESAT-6-like antigen identified in the highly virulent *Mycobacterium tuberculosis* Beijing K strain. Frontiers in Microbiology. 2019;**10**:220. DOI: 10.3389/fmicb.2019.00220

[89] World Health Organisation: WHO Director-General declares the ongoing Monkeypox outbreak a Public Health Emergency of International Concern. Available from: https://www.who.int/europe/news/item/23-07-2022-who-director-general-declares-the-ongoing-monkeypox-outbreak-a-public-health-event-of-international-concern [Accessed: July 25, 2022]

[90] Maxmen A. Unseating big pharma: The radical plan for vaccine equity. Nature. 2022;**607**(7918):226-233. DOI: 10.1038/d41586-022-01898-3

[91] Mandala WL, Liu MKP. SARS-CoV-2 and HIV-1: Should HIV-1-infected individuals in sub-Saharan Africa Be considered a priority group for the COVID-19 vaccines? Frontiers in Immunology. 2021;**12**:797117. DOI: 10.3389/fimmu.2021.797117

Chapter 7

Outer Membrane Vesicles: A Challenging Yet Promising Platform for COVID-19 Vaccines

Amanda Izeli Portilho and Elizabeth De Gaspari

Abstract

The outer membrane vesicles (OMVs) are vesicles released from Gram-negative bacteria, which present a range of biological applications, such as vaccine adjuvants. OMVs present several pathogen-associated molecular patterns, being immunogenic and capable of triggering different arms of the immune response. Thus, they are suitable for mucosal and parenteral delivery, feasible to obtain and have been used in licensed-vaccines previously. However, the extraction protocols and manipulations can modify OMVs cargo and, consequentially, the immunization results. Therefore, this chapter will review OMVs use as adjuvant and discuss results from COVID-19 vaccines which employed this technique.

Keywords: COVID-19, outer membrane vesicles, SARS-CoV-2, adjuvants

1. Introduction

Outer membrane vesicles (OMVs) are naturally released vesicles from the outer membrane of Gram-negative bacteria. These vesicles are composed by several antigens, such as lipopolysaccharide (LPS), phospholipids, and specific proteins, according to the bacterium species [1], hence, being important for bacteria evolution and survival [2]. The antigens of OMVs also act as pathogen-associated molecular patterns (PAMPs), and their use as vaccine adjuvants have been discussed [3]. OMVs not only activate innate immunity but also improve humoral and cellular adaptative responses, and they are affordable to obtain and suitable for different immunization routes—parenteral and mucosal. OMVs vaccines against *Neisseria meningitidis*, a Gram-negative pathogen, have already been approved for human use [4].

The COVID-19 pandemic led to an urge for vaccines. To address this issue, different vaccine platforms have been tested and developed in record time [5, 6]. It is crucial that all countries have access to vaccines to control the disease [7]. Local production supports this universal access, provided that it diminishes the costs of vaccine manufacturing compared to commercial values; thus, it facilitates the distribution [8]. However, the local production should be suitable to infrastructure, expertise, and other particularities of each country [9].

Adjuvants are used to improve vaccine efficacy—they increase the antigen's immunogenicity, support dose sparing, and modulate the overall immunity toward

 IntechOpen

an adequate pattern of response [10]. This chapter aims to describe OMVs structure, explain their adjuvant effect, and discuss how they could be used for COVID-19 vaccines.

2. Outer membrane vesicles: biology, isolation, and purification

OMVs are negative-charged circular structures, ranging from 20 to 250 nm, produced through the blebbing of the outer membrane of Gram-negative bacteria [3]. This outer membrane is composed of a phospholipid bilayer, expressing lipopolysaccharide (LPS, or endotoxin) and several other antigens, depending on the bacterium species and strain. Below the outer membrane, there is a layer of peptidoglycan and the inner membrane [11].

To release the vesicles, the outer membrane is detached from the peptidoglycan; however, bacterium integrity must be preserved. This process is mediated by cross-linking proteins and lipids: such molecules are expressed in the outer membrane and linked with peptidoglycan, so the modulation of these molecules might increase or decrease the membranes' attachment [11]. The outer membrane protein A (OmpA) protein, the Tol-Pal complex, and the LPS are examples of cross-linking molecules related to OMV release [12, 13].

The bacterium modulates OMV release to cover different functions: communication between bacteria; transportation of protein, DNA or RNA; metabolites excretion; nutrient acquisition; protection against bacteriophages and biofilm production, among others [1]. **Figure 1** shows the organization of a Gram-negative bacterium envelope, the blebbing of the outer membrane, and summarizes the functions of these structures.

Even though the OMVs are produced physiologically by bacterium, the isolation of these structures following natural release provides a limited number of vesicles.

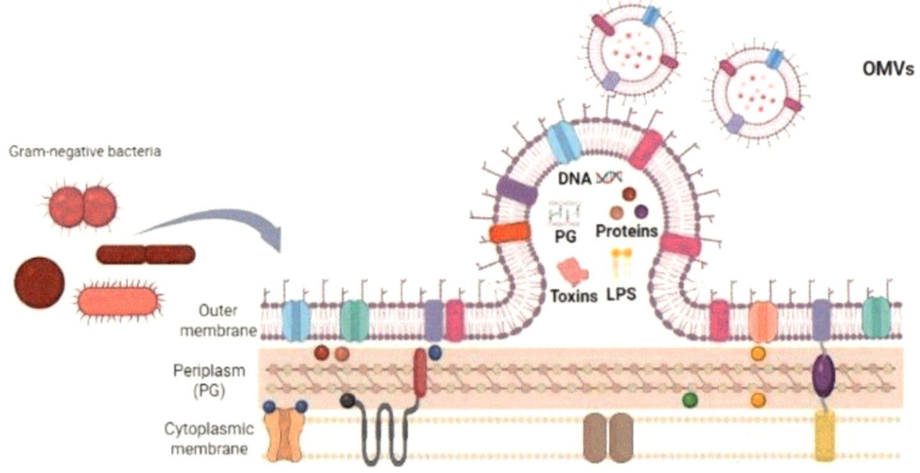

Figure 1.
Structure, release, and content of OMVs: Gram-negative bacteria present a complex cell wall, formed by a cytoplasmic membrane, the periplasm, which has a thin peptidoglycan layer and the outer membrane. The membranes are composed of a phospholipid bilayer and present LPS, among other antigens (according to the bacterium strain). The vesicles originate from the blebbing of the outer membrane and carry various structures, such as the LPS, proteins, DNA, and toxins, which are capable of activating the immune system. OMVs: outer membrane vesicles, LPS: lipopolysaccharide, PG: peptidoglycan. (Figure created with BioRender).

Hence, laboratory protocols were standardized to improve OMVs induction [2]. The first techniques consisted of chemical protocols to put the cells under stressful conditions, modulating pH and molarity through detergents and salts [14]. With the popularization of genetic engineering, it became possible to manipulate the bacterium strains to release more vesicles [15]. Moreover, the molecular approach allows to overexpress antigens of interest in the OMVs content [2].

Another application of genetically modified OMVs was developed by GlaxoSmithKline. The generalized modules for membrane antigens (GMMAs) are OMVs obtained by Gram-negative bacteria engineered to improve vesiculation [16]. A *Shigella* vaccine developed using this strategy entered clinical trials [17]. Nevertheless, this strategy is versatile, since antigens from different pathogens can be coupled to the OMVs—*Mycobacterium tuberculosis* and *Chlamydia trachomatis* were proven to work—exploring vesicles as delivery and adjuvant system combined [16, 18].

Given that Gram-negative bacteria express LPS, which is highly reactogenic, this antigen should be purified from the OMVs, respecting the acceptable levels for preclinical and clinical trials [19]. This is the reason that led to the popularization of deoxycholate extraction—the detergent stimulates OMV release and reduces the LPS content concomitantly [1]. When different protocols are used to produce OMVs, the LPS detoxification can be performed using Sepharose-4B-Polymyxin or monoclonal antibodies columns [20]. Recently, a removal protocol using Cationic amphiphilic peptides was proposed [21]. Another option is to use bioengineered strains, modified to express a nontoxic LPS [22].

Finally, it is important to understand that different protocols result in different OMV content. The ideal OMV composition for the planned application should be aligned with the extraction method [23].

3. Outer membrane vesicles and immune activation

OMVs were firstly used for pathogen-specific vaccines against *Neisseria meningitidis* from serogroup B [4]. However, antigens present in OMVs cargo, regardless of bacteria species, act as pathogen-associated molecular patterns (PAMPs). With the increasing understanding about the interplay between innate and adaptative immunity, PAMPs have been suggested as promising adjuvants [9].

Several pattern recognition receptors (PRRs) recognize OMVs structures. Considering the Toll-like receptors (TLRs) family, Flagellin activates TLR-5, CpG DNA is recognized by TLR-9, ribosomal RNA activates TLR-13, and other lipoproteins can interact with TLRs-1, -2, and -6 [3]. LPS binds to TLR-4, although, as discussed previously, its concentration should be under acceptable levels for clinical use [19]. In addition, OMVs from bacteria like *Aggregatibacter actinomycetemcomitans* and *Escherichia coli* activated NOD-(NOD) like receptors in cell culture [24, 25]. *Bordetella pertussis* vesicles upregulated the NLRP3 inflammasome pathway [26]. The outer membrane protein A (OmpA) from *Klebsiella pneumonia* was described as an activator of innate and humoral responses interacting with scavenger receptors LOX-1 and SREC, TLR-2, and long pentraxin PTX-3 [27].

Not only PRRs are activated, but different immune pathways could be explored using OMVs as adjuvants. The vesicles of *Moxarella catarrhalis* and *Haemophilus influenzae* activated B-cells via IgD receptor [28, 29]. B-cell-independent activation is not the main goal of vaccination, since a T-cell-dependent response is needed for immunologic memory. However, OMVs also support T-cell activation and B-cell proliferation [30].

OMVs from *B. pertussis* supported cellular and humoral immune response of the mucosa, upregulating genes related to Th17 response and IgA secretion [31].

Importantly, it was verified that preexisting immunity against the vesicles did not affect the adjuvanticity potential [32]. Besides that, the 20–250 nm size of OMVs is ideal for uptake by antigen-presenting cells (APCs) and OMVs upregulate genes related to antigen presentation molecules, such as CD-80, CD-86, and MHC-II in macrophages and dendritic cells [3, 30]. All that considered, the immune activation conferred by OMVs makes them an interesting adjuvant [2].

Noteworthy, activating PRRs triggers cellular signaling that culminates in an inflammatory response [9]. Because of that, the reactogenicity of OMVs should be studied. Rossi et al. [33] reviewed the tests available (such as rabbit pyrogenicity and monocyte activation tests) and their advantages and limitations.

To note, Gram-positive bacteria also release membrane vesicles; however, only recently the scientific community has started to investigate them. Vesicles of *Mycobacterium* genus are known to activate TLR-2, and extracellular vesicles of *Streptococcus pneumoniae* and *Bacillus anthracis* were effective antigens for immunization against these pathogens [34]. Vesicles isolated from *Streptococcus pneumoniae* were internalized by dendritic cells and enhanced tumor necrosis factor (TNF)-α release, without toxic effects [35]. The use of such vesicles as adjuvants might be a promising field of study too.

4. Previous experience using OMVs in vaccines

The OMVs were first studied as a technology to develop vaccines against *N. meningitidis* from serogroup B. During the 80s, three OMV-based vaccines were used to control meningococcal disease epidemics: Va-Mengoc-BC (Finlay Institute) in Cuba, MENZB (Novartis) in New Zealand and MenBvac (Norwegian Institute of Public Health) in Norway [4].

Recent efforts to develop an OMV vaccine against *Shigella sonnei* were undertaken, as well as to use *N. meningitidis* OMV vaccines to prevent *N. gonorrhoeae* infection [36, 37]. Supported by the success of the *S. sonnei* OMV vaccine,

Vaccine	Pathogen	Phase	Reference(s)
Va-Mengoc-BC (Finlay Institute)	*N. meningitidis*	Licensed	[4]
MENZB (Novartis)	*N. meningitidis*	Licensed	[4]
MenBvac (Norwegian Institute of Public Health)	*N. meningitidis*	Licensed	[4]
S. sonnei GMMA (1790GAHB) (GlaxoSmithKline)	*S. sonnei*	Phase I	[17]
S. Typhimurium GMMA (GlaxoSmithKline)	*S.* Typhimurium	Entering Phase I/II	[16]
S. Enteritidis GMMA (GlaxoSmithKline)	*S.* Enteritidis	Entering Phase I/II	[16]
Soberana 01 (Finlay Institute)	SARS-CoV-2	Phase II clinical trial	[38, 39]

Table 1.
OMV-based vaccines licensed or in clinical trials against different pathogens.

GlaxoSmithKline is about to start clinical trials using the same platform for *Salmonella* vaccines [16]. OMVs seem an interesting platform for *B. pertussis* vaccines as well, although no candidates went to clinical trials yet [2]. **Table 1** summarizes the OMVs-based vaccines which have been studied in clinical trials. The Soberana 01, a COVID-19 vaccine which uses OMVs as adjuvant, will be discussed in more detail in the next section.

Nonetheless, OMVs are immunogenic, stable, and feasible to isolate, making them an affordable vaccine platform and adjuvant option [9].

5. COVID-19 vaccines and outer membrane vesicles: promising results

The importance of affordable, accessible vaccines has been highlighted since the beginning of the COVID-19 pandemic [40]. As discussed so far, the vesicles are feasible to obtain, are immunogenic, improve the humoral and cellular arms of the immune response, and are suitable for both parenteral and mucosal delivery [2]. Thus, OMVs have been licensed for human use before [4].

Before SARS-CoV-2, OMVs were explored as vaccine adjuvants for other viruses. A fusion of Zika virus and *N. meningitidis* OMVs resulted in a promising nanoparticle, which enhanced IgG titers, cytokine markers of Th1/Th2 responses, and immunologic memory, such as IL-2/IL-4 and TGF-β. Moreover, the nanoparticles induced neutralizing antibodies against the Zika virus when administrated alone or combined with mesoporous silica as adjuvant [41].

Different investigations proposed OMVs of *E. coli* as Influenza adjuvant. In Shim et al. Alum and an oil-in-water emulsion were more effective to enhance the antibody titers, but OMVs modulated the immune response toward a Th1 profile, with IFN-γ and higher IgG2c/IgG1 ratio; thus, the hemagglutinin inhibition titers were higher using OMVs as adjuvants. All that resulted in protection of ferrets after a lethal viral challenge [42]. Watkins et al. also used OMVs as Influenza adjuvant. Similarly, the immunization resulted in the survival of mice from different genetic backgrounds after lethal viral challenges using H1N1 and H3N2 viruses. Thus, the humoral response presented a mixed Th1/Th2 profile. Interestingly, the authors observed that the OMVs promoted DCs activation and maturation, even though they expressed a modified LPS with reduced reactogenicity [43].

A multivalent Influenza/Middle East Respiratory Syndrome Coronavirus (MERS-CoV) vaccine adjuvanted was recently proposed. OMVs from *E. coli* presenting the hemagglutinin of Influenza H1N1 and the receptor-binding domain (RBD) of MERS-CoV induced neutralizing antibodies against both viruses and immunized animals survived an H1N1 challenge [44]. Taken together, these results show that OMVs are a versatile tool to adjuvant heterologous antigens, even in multivalent strategies.

The COVID-19 vaccine database of the World Health Organization (WHO) (updated on July 22, 2022) describes two vaccines using OMVs in preclinical trials. Plus, Soberana 01, from Finlay Institute, uses OMVs as adjuvants and is going into Phase II trials [38, 45]. Even though this is an unexpressive number, promising results were obtained in preclinical experiments.

The receptor binding domain (RBD) of SARS-CoV-2, adjuvanted by OMVs from *N. meningitidis* (from serogroups B or C) and Alum, improved IgA and IgG titers, thus, IL-1 and IL-17 secretion following a mixed intramuscular/intranasal delivery [46]. Besides that, the adjuvants contributed to increasing avidity and neutralization of antibodies [47], which are relevant parameters for COVID-19 humoral response [48].

Similarly, the Spike protein adjuvanted by OMVs from *N. meningitidis* induced a robust humoral response, with neutralizing antibodies and prevention of viral replication after challenge [49]. To note, the intranasal delivery of the antigenic preparation induced IgA in the nose and the lungs, conferring mucosal protection [49].

Vibrio cholerae and *E. coli* OMVs were compared as adjuvants for intranasal RBD immunization [50]. Both preparations elicited a robust systemic and mucosal immune response, supported by neutralizing antibodies. The most promising results were obtained when OMVs from each bacterium were administrated in turn, as a heterogeneous prime-booster approach [50].

An intranasal vaccine composed of the Spike protein and OMVs from *Salmonella typhimurium* induced not only systemic and mucosal immunity but also neutralizing antibodies against the delta variant. Upon viral challenge, only hamsters immunized with the adjuvanted preparation presented less severe lung pathology and lower virus titers in bronchoalveolar lavage [51].

The Finlay Institute responded to the pandemic developing Soberana 01, which uses RBD as antigen and vesicles from *N. meningitidis* from serogroup B and alum as adjuvants. In mice, they observed that this formulation was more immunogenic than RBD only adsorbed in Alum: it induced robust B-cell memory and neutralizing antibodies; thus, the antibodies recognized mutant RBD from SARS-CoV-2 variants [39]. Considering clinical use, the group described that the vaccine was safe and immunogenic, and the OMVs contributed to inducing functional, neutralizing antibodies [45].

6. Conclusion

In conclusion, OMVs are versatile tools with several biological applications, including vaccine development. The adjuvanticity of these vesicles relies on the innate immunity activation conferred by PAMPs; however, OMVs expression changes according to bacterium species and extraction protocol. OMVs are stable, safe, and suitable for mucosal and parenteral delivery. In addition, having a history of previous use in vaccines makes them a promising adjuvant candidate for translating to clinical use. Preclinical data showed that OMVs supported functional antibodies and protection against SARS-CoV-2; thus, there are COVID-19 vaccines adjuvanted by OMVs undergoing clinical trials. Nonetheless, OMVs prove how biomolecules produced by microorganisms are remarkable tools for the biomedical area.

Acknowledgements

This chapter was supported by São Paulo Research Foundation (FAPESP) (grant number 18/04202-0) and Coordination for the Improvement of Higher Education Personnel (grant number 88887.661236/2022-00).

Conflict of interest

The authors declare no conflict of interest.

Author details

Amanda Izeli Portilho[1,2] and Elizabeth De Gaspari[1,2]*

1 Immunology Center, Adolfo Lutz Institute, São Paulo, Brazil

2 Graduate Program Interunits in Biotechnology, University of São Paulo, São Paulo, Brazil

*Address all correspondence to: elizabeth.gaspari@ial.sp.gov.br

References

[1] Acevedo R, Fernández S, Zayas C, Acosta A, Sarmiento ME, Ferro VA, et al. Bacterial outer membrane vesicles and vaccine applications. Frontiers in Immunology. 2014;**5**:1-6

[2] Balhuizen MD, Veldhuizen EJA, Haagsman HP. Outer membrane vesicle induction and isolation for vaccine development. Frontiers in Microbiology. 2021;**12**:629090

[3] Mancini F, Rossi O, Necchi F, Micoli F. OMV vaccines and the role of TLR agonists in immune response. International Journal of Molecular Sciences. 2020;**21**:1-19

[4] Pizza M, Bekkat-Berkani R, Rappuoli R. Vaccines against meningococcal diseases. Microorganisms. 2020;**8**:1-21

[5] Forni G, Mantovani A, Forni G, Mantovani A, Moretta L, Rappuoli R, et al. COVID-19 vaccines: Where we stand and challenges ahead. Cell Death and Differentiation. 2021;**28**:626-639

[6] Chong WC, Chellappan DK, Shukla SD, Peterson GM, Patel RP, Jha NK, et al. An appraisal of the current scenario in vaccine research for COVID-19. Viruses. 2021;**13**:1-18

[7] Blumental S, Debré P. Challenges and Issues of Anti-SARS-CoV-2 Vaccines. Frontiers in Medicine. 2021;**8**:1-11

[8] Munira SL, Hendriks JT, Atmosukarto II, Friede MH, Carter LM, Butler JRG, et al. A cost analysis of producing vaccines in developing countries. Vaccine. 2019;**37**:1245-1251

[9] Miyaji EN, Carvalho E, Oliveira MLS, Raw I, Ho PL. Trends in adjuvant development for vaccines: DAMPs and PAMPs as potential new adjuvants. Brazilian Journal of Medical and Biological Research. 2011;**44**:500-513

[10] Savelkoul HFJ, Ferro VA, Strioga MM, Schijns VEJC. Choice and design of adjuvants for parenteral and mucosal vaccines. Vaccine. 2015;**3**:148-171

[11] Schwechheimer C, Kuehn MJ. Outer-membrane vesicles from Gram-negative bacteria: Biogenesis and functions. Nature Reviews. Microbiology. 2015;**13**:605-619

[12] Cascales E, Bernadac A, Gavioli M, Lazzaroni JC, Lloubes R. Pal lipoprotein of *Escherichia coli* plays a major role in outer membrane integrity. Journal of Bacteriology. 2002;**184**:754-759

[13] Avila-Calderón ED et al. Outer membrane vesicles of gram-negative bacteria: An outlook on biogenesis. Frontiers in Microbiology. 2021;**12**:557902

[14] Frasch CE, Peppler MS. Protection against group B *Neisseria meningitidis* disease: Preparation of soluble protein and protein-polysaccharide immunogens. Infection and Immunity. 1982;**37**:271-280

[15] van de Waterbeemd B, Streefland M, van der Ley P, Zomer B, van Dijken H, Martens D, et al. Improved OMV vaccine against *Neisseria meningitidis* using genetically engineered strains and a detergent-free purification process. Vaccine. 2010;**28**:4810-4816

[16] Mancini F, Micoli F, Necchi F, Pizza M, Berlanda Scorza F, Rossi O. GMMA-based vaccines: The known and the unknown. Frontiers in Immunology. 2021;**12**:1-7

[17] Launay O, Lewis DJM, Anemona A, Loulergue P, Leahy J, Sciré AS, et al. Safety profile and immunologic responses of a novel vaccine against *Shigella sonnei* administered intramuscularly, intradermally and intranasally: Results from two parallel randomized Phase 1 Clinical Studies in Healthy Adult Volunteers in Europe. eBioMedicine. 2017;**22**:164-172

[18] Daleke-Schermerhorn MH, Felix T, Soprova Z, ten Hagen-Jongman CM, Vikström D, Majlessi L, et al. Decoration of outer membrane vesicles with multiple antigens by using an autotransporter approach. Applied and Environmental Microbiology. 2014;**80**:5854-5865

[19] Brito LA, Singh M. Acceptable levels of Endotoxin in vaccine formulations during preclinical research. Journal of Pharmaceutical Sciences. 2011;**100**:34-37

[20] Magalhães PO, Lopes AM, Mazzola PG, Rangel-Yagui C, Penna TCV, Pessoa A Jr. Methods of endotoxin removal from biological preparations: A review. Journal of Pharmaceutical Sciences. 2011;**10**:1-15

[21] Sepahi M, Hadadian S, Ahangari CohanR, NorouzianD. Lipopolysaccharide removal affinity matrices based on novel cationic amphiphilic peptides. Preparative Biochemistry & Biotechnology. 2021;**51**:386-394

[22] Kim SH, Kim KS, Lee SR, Kim E, Kim MS, Lee EY, et al. Structural modifications of outer membrane vesicles to refine them as vaccine delivery vehicles. Biochimica et Biophysica Acta, Biomembranes. 1788;**2009**:2150-2159

[23] van der Pol L, Stork M, van der Ley P. Outer membrane vesicles as platform vaccine technology. Biotechnology Journal. 2015;**10**:1689-1706

[24] Thay B, Damm A, Kufer TA, Wai SN, Oscarsson J. *Aggregatibacter actinomycetemcomitans* outer membrane vesicles are internalized in human host cells and trigger NOD1- and NOD2-dependent NF-κB activation. Infection and Immunity. 2014;**82**:4034-4046

[25] Cañas MA, Fábrega MJ, Giménez R, Badia J, Baldomà L. Outer membrane vesicles from probiotic and commensal *Escherichia coli* activate NOD1-mediated immune responses in intestinal epithelial cells. Frontiers in Microbiology. 2018;**9**:1-13

[26] Elizagaray ML, Gomes MTR, Guimaraes ES, Rumbo M, Hozbor DF, Oliveira SC, et al. Canonical and non-canonical inflammasome activation by outer membrane vesicles derived from *Bordetella pertussis*. Frontiers in Immunology. 2020;**11**:1-13

[27] Jeannin P, Bottazzi B, Sironi M, Doni A, Rusnati M, Presta M, et al. Complexity and complementarity of outer membrane protein A recognition by cellular and humoral innate immunity receptors. Immunity. 2005;**22**:551-560

[28] Deknuydt F, Nordström T, Riesbeck K. Diversion of the host humoral response: A novel virulence mechanism of *Haemophilus influenzae* mediated via outer membrane vesicles. Journal of Leukocyte Biology. 2014;**95**:983-991

[29] Perez Vidakovics MLA, Jendholm J, Mörgelin M, Månsson A, Larsson C, Cardell LO, et al. B cell activation by outer membrane vesicles - A novel virulence mechanism. PLoS Pathogens. 2010;**6**:e1000724

[30] Cai W, Kesavan DK, Wan J, Abdelaziz MH, Su Z, Xu H. Bacterial outer membrane vesicles, a potential vaccine candidate in interactions with

host cells based. Diagnostic Pathology. 2018;**13**:1-12

[31] Raeven RHM, Brummelman J, Pennings J La, Van Der Maas L, Helm K, Tilstra W, et al. Molecular and cellular signatures underlying superior immunity against *Bordetella pertussis* upon pulmonary vaccination. Mucosal Immunology 2018;11:979-993.

[32] Timothy Prior J, Davitt C, Kurtz J, Gellings P, McLachlan JB, Morici LA. Bacterial-derived outer membrane vesicles are potent adjuvants that drive humoral and cellular immune responses. Pharmaceutics. 2021;**13**:1-11

[33] Rossi O, Citiulo F, Mancini F. Outer membrane vesicles: Moving within the intricate labyrinth of assays that can predict risks of reactogenicity in humans. Human Vaccines & Immunotherapeutics. 2020;**17**:1-13

[34] Brown L, Wolf JM, Prados-Rosales R, Casadevall A. Through the wall: Extracellular vesicles in Gram-positive bacteria, mycobacteria and fungi. Nature Reviews. Microbiology. 2015;**13**:620-630

[35] Mehanny M, Koch M, Lehr CM, Fuhrmann G. Streptococcal extracellular membrane vesicles are rapidly internalized by immune cells and alter their cytokine release. Frontiers in Immunology. 2020;**11**:1-13

[36] Micoli F, MacLennan CA. Outer membrane vesicle vaccines. Seminars in Immunology. 2020;**50**:101433

[37] Semchenko EA, Seib KL. Outer membrane vesicle vaccines for *Neisseria gonorrhoeae*. Nature Reviews. Urology. 2022;**19**:5-6

[38] World Health Organization. COVID-19 vaccine tracker and landscape 2022. 2022. https://www.who.int/publications/m/item/draft-landscape-of-covid-19-candidate-vaccines. [Accessed February 9, 2022]

[39] Santana-Mederos D, Perez-Nicado R, Climent Y, Rodriguez L, Ramirez BS, Perez-Rodriguez S, et al. A COVID-19 vaccine candidate composed of the SARS-CoV-2 RBD dimer and *Neisseria meningitidis* outer membrane vesicles. RSC Chem Biol. 2022;**3**:242-249

[40] Forman R, Anderson M, Jit M, Mossialos E. Ensuring access and affordability through COVID-19 vaccine research and development investments: A proposal for the options market for vaccines. Vaccine. 2020;**38**:6075-6077

[41] Martins P, Machado D, Theizen TH, Guarnieri JPO, Bernardes BG, Gomide GP, et al. Outer membrane vesicles from *Neisseria meningitidis* (proteossome) used for nanostructured Zika virus vaccine production. Scientific Reports. 2018;**8**:1-10

[42] Shim SM, Song EJ, Song D, Lee TY, Kim DJ, Nam JH, et al. Nontoxic outer membrane vesicles efficiently increase the efficacy of an influenza vaccine in mice and ferrets. Vaccine. 2017;**35**:3741-3748

[43] Watkins HC, Rappazzo CG, Higgins JS, Sun X, Brock N, Chau A, et al. Safe recombinant outer membrane vesicles that display M2e elicit heterologous influenza protection. Molecular Therapy. 2017;**25**:989-1002

[44] Shehata MM, Mostafa A, Teubner L, Mahmoud SH, Kandeil A, Elshesheny R, et al. Bacterial outer membrane vesicles (OMVs)-based dual vaccine for influenza a H1N1 virus and MERS-CoV. Vaccine. 2019;7:1-13

[45] Pérez-RodríguezS,delaCaridadR-GM, Ochoa-Azze R, Climent-Ruiz Y, Alberto

González-Delgado C, Paredes-Moreno B, et al. A randomized, double-blind phase I clinical trial of two recombinant dimeric RBD COVID-19 vaccine candidates: Safety, reactogenicity and immunogenicity. Vaccine. 2022;**40**:2068-2075

[46] Gaspar EB, Prudencio CR, De Gaspari E. Experimental studies using OMV in a new platform of SARS-CoV-2 vaccines. Human Vaccines & Immunotherapeutics. 2021;**17**: 2965-2968

[47] Gaspar EB, De Gaspari E. Avidity assay to test functionality of anti-SARS-CoV-2 antibodies. Vaccine. 2021;**39**:1473-1475

[48] Bauer G. High avidity of vaccine-induced immunoglobulin G against SARS-CoV-2: Potential relevance for protective humoral immunity. Exploration of Immunology. 2022;**2**: 133-156

[49] van der Ley PA, Zariri A, van Riet E, Oosterhoff D, Kruiswijk CP. An intranasal OMV-based vaccine induces high mucosal and systemic protecting immunity against a SARS-CoV-2 infection. Frontiers in Immunology. 2021;**12**:1-11

[50] Thapa HB, Müller AM, Camilli A, Schild S. An intranasal vaccine based on outer membrane vesicles against SARS-CoV-2. Frontiers in Microbiology. 2021;**12**:1-16

[51] Jiang L, Driedonks TAP, Jong WSP, Dhakal S, Bart van den Berg van Saparoea H, Sitaras I, et al. A bacterial extracellular vesicle-based intranasal vaccine against SARS-CoV-2 protects against disease and elicits neutralizing antibodies to wild-type and Delta variants. Journal of Extracellular Vesicles. 2022;**11**:e12192

Chapter 8

Repurposing BCG and MMR Vaccines for Combating COVID-19: A Review and Opinion Based on Clinical Evidence

Kasturi Mahesh Tawde, Aditya Manivannan Iyer and Harshal Ashok Pawar

Abstract

Our review comprehends past and recent developments encircling the two vaccines, BCG and MMR, which have efficacy lasting 10 years and are known to trigger the production of Interferon and various cytokines. BCG has depicted long-lasting effects, reduction in mortality, and hospitalizations associated with various diseases in different age groups as per studies across Sweden, West Africa, Spain, and Indonesia. Clinical trials are in progress in Holland, Australia, and Germany to study its effects on COVID-19. Most Asian countries with childhood BCG vaccination programs have shown lower COVID-19-related per capita death rates. The MMR vaccination has shown a reduction in hospitalizations and COVID-19-related deaths in about 11 countries, and a randomized clinical trial has been proposed in New Orleans. Reasons such as inhibition of pulmonary inflammation and structural similarity have been cited for such consequences. BCG and MMR may serve to shorten the duration of infection, minimize harmful pathology, reduce hospitalization rates, and curb the spread of the disease, but more research is required to assess the associated risks, especially for the elderly and people with comorbidities who are prone to severe complications of COVID-19.

Keywords: BCG, MMR, COVID-19, vaccines, SARS-CoV-2, coronavirus

1. Introduction

Ever since the coronavirus disease (COVID-19) emerged, there has been an onset in development of multiple vaccine candidates across the globe. On the one hand, scientists are developing specific vaccines, while on the other hand, existing vaccines are getting explored for repositioning. The latter offers to reduce the overall cost and time.

The novel coronavirus SARS-CoV-2 disease was reported in Wuhan, and the underlying causative agent was found to belong to the family *Coronaviridae* [1, 2]. Human-to-human transmission via physical contact and respiratory droplets when an infected individual coughs or sneezes is preventable via strategies such as social distancing and maintenance of hygiene [1, 3]. The virus comprises a single-stranded, positive-sense RNA genome containing 29,903 nucleotides. Orf1ab gene encodes nonstructural proteins. Some genes encode structural proteins, some of which include spike (S), membrane (M), nucleocapsid (N), and envelope (E) while other genes encode the accessory proteins such as orf3a, orf6, orf7, and orf10 [1, 2].

The disease has been progressing for a while now. Although there is a cut-throat race among nations to launch their vaccine candidates, there is a lot underway that is meant to prove each candidate's safety, efficacy, and superiority over the other. The vaccine candidates are in various stages of development. Whereas a vaccine usually takes years to reach a market, vaccine development has increased in speed in recent times. In such moments of immense vigor to be ahead in the race, there are two non-specific vaccine candidates, Bacillus Calmette-Guérin (BCG) and Measles, Mumps, and Rubella (MMR) vaccine, which appear promising.

The popular BCG and MMR vaccines confer broad immunity against diseases not limited to tuberculosis (TB) and measles, mumps, and rubella. Substantial clinical and nonclinical evidence proves their nonspecific nature alongside their safety and efficacy. With such time constraints, they could stand a chance to be candidates to combat COVID-19. The study thus compares and comprehends the practicality of the two vaccine candidates, giving them the basis of global clinical evidence, underlying mechanisms of immunity conferment, and their current prospects to test whether they stand a chance in combating COVID-19.

2. Bacillus Calmette-Guérin (BCG) vaccine

The Bacillus Calmette-Guérin (BCG) is a renowned vaccine known to confer prevention and cross-protection against *Mycobacterium tuberculosis* infection. It is composed of *Mycobacterium bovis* in the attenuated form [4, 5]. This vaccine was first used on humans in 1921 [6]. BCG vaccination of newborns and infants reduces the risk of pulmonary TB by about 50% [7], and it is administered in infants intradermally post-birth [1]. Nearly 100 million newborns are administered the BCG vaccine annually [5]. It is protective in young children previously not infected by the severe forms of tuberculosis [8]. Although it has shown clear protection in children, its effects have been inconsistent in adults [9].

BCG vaccination has broad protective effects that are not specific to *Mycobacterium tuberculosis* infection, which has been proven with sufficient evidence.

2.1 Clinical evidence for broad protective effects against COVID-19

In 1927, Swedish children who were administered the BCG vaccine at birth showed a mortality rate almost threefold lower than the unvaccinated children [10]. On similar grounds, a BCG vaccination scar and a positive tuberculin reaction conferred better survival during early childhood in an area with high mortality in West Africa [11]. The long-lasting effect of BCG was recognized in a study based in Spain, wherein the hospitalizations associated with respiratory infections other than TB in 0–14-year-old children were found to be substantially lower in BCG-vaccinated children. This protection in 14-year-olds confirmed the enduring broad protective effect of BCG [12]. Two separate randomized human clinical trials are being conducted to test the prospect and likeliness of its conferment of protection against COVID-19. These are in progress in Holland [1, 13] and Australia [1, 14]. In these studies, health workers are being administered either the BCG vaccine or a placebo saline injection. A small study in Indonesia found that vaccination of adults in the age group of 60–75 years with BCG prevented acute upper respiratory tract infections by an increase in IFN-γ levels. The study involved the administration of the BCG vaccine once every month for 3 months. The placebo group received solvent for the BCG vaccine [15].

There is a possibility that the innate immune response to vaccination depends on the strain of BCG and the route of administration. Even short-span protection may help individuals at high risk, such as front-line workers, until there is the availability of a specific vaccine. Most Asian countries have active universal BCG vaccination programs. However, with no direct evidence from clinical trials, it is not yet advisable to recommend the use of BCG to prevent COVID-19.

A report found the presence of a strong correlation between the BCG index and COVID-19 mortality in European countries. The index is an estimation of the degree of universal BCG vaccination deployment in a given country. With every 10% increase in this index, there was a 10.4% reduction in mortality associated with COVID-19 [16].

2.2 Basis of broad protective effects against COVID-19

Clinical and laboratory experimental evidence suggests prevention against viral infections in humans [17]. Trained immunity and long-lasting protection from the respiratory tract's viral infections are offered by BCG vaccination, which eventually becomes a basis for its potential protective effect against COVID-19 [16].

Prevention of vaccinia virus infection is conferred via an enhancement in interferon-gamma production (IFN-γ) from CD4+ cells in BCG-vaccinated mice [18], which is attributed to adaptive immunity. There is a rise in levels of pro-inflammatory cytokines such as Interleukin-1β (IL-1β) involved in immunity against viruses [19]. Interleukin-2 (IL-2), TNF-α (tumor necrosis factor), and IFN-γ (interferon- γ) are released because of the activation of CD4+ T cells [20].

T-helper cells are activated once BCG gets internalized by antigen-presenting cells. MHC class II molecules expressed on the surface of APCs and recognized by the CD4+ T cells via the T-cell receptor (TCR) bring about this activation. This interaction between MHC II molecules and TCR is governed by the binding of co-stimulatory molecules (CD28) to B7–1 on the T cells, and this binding causes an upregulation of adhesion molecules such as LFA-1 (lymphocytes function associated antigens-1). The LFA-1 binds to the macrophages via ICAM-1 (intracellular adhesion molecule-1) [21].

There is evidence for the conferment of immunity against listeria and influenza in murine models [22, 23]. Various controlled trials have shown that BCG vaccination reduces the severity of infections by several viruses with structural similarity to SARS-CoV-2 [1].

In 2015, a placebo-controlled randomized trial revealed that the immunogenicity of the H1N1 vaccine was augmented in healthy adults because of BCG vaccination [24].

2.3 The current status

At present, three active ongoing advancing clinical trials are examining whether the BCG vaccination prevents SARS-CoV-2 infection in healthcare workers [1].

Currently, the World Health Organization (WHO) does not recommend using the BCG vaccine to cope with COVID-19 as there is no firm evidence suggesting prevention of the SARS-CoV-2 infection [25]. Whether the BCG vaccine administered decades ago in childhood will prevent or treat COVID-19 now is debatable [1]. There is a possibility that the BCG vaccine may upregulate the immune system, aggravating the severity of COVID-19 in a few patients. Its supply is already low, and a false sense of security might mislead the population, eventually compromising the fulfillment of the needs of infants for protection against tuberculosis in high-risk zones [26, 27].

Japan, China, Korea, India, and the Russian Federation have continued to conduct childhood BCG vaccination. Compared with the countries with no mandatory mass BCG vaccination, the per capita death rate associated with COVID-19 in the countries mentioned above is lower. Japan, Brazil, and Russia incorporate BCG vaccines containing original strains compared with the European countries where the vaccine contains modified strains [28].

A team is conducting a study at the Max Planck Institute for Infection Biology in Germany to test whether VPM1002, a recombinant BCG vaccine strain, can protect healthcare workers or older patients from COVID-19 [28–30].

The cause-and-effect relationship between the BCG vaccine and COVID-19 is yet to be proven with concrete evidence. There is a limitation associated with the above understandings. In low-income countries where there could be reduced testing capabilities, substantial under-reporting of the number of cases and deaths may undermine the possibility of getting an exact correlation between COVID-19-related mortality and BCG [31]. Although it appears as if the countries without mandatory mass BCG vaccination policies [32], such as the United States and Italy, have higher mortality rates, there may be a dependence of mortality rate associated with COVID-19 [16] on factors such as temperature, percentage of population 65 years or older in a particular region, GDP, population density, and its variation from state to state.

There is a lack of mandatory vaccination programs in countries such as the United States, Canada, Italy, and the Netherlands [32]. The vaccine is administered at birth and offers protection against tuberculosis for 10 years [5].

3. Measles, mumps, and rubella (MMR) vaccine

The Measles, Mumps, and Rubella (MMR) vaccine is a combination vaccine used to confer immunity against measles, mumps, and rubella infections [33]. This live attenuated multi-dose vaccine [34] possesses various combinations of strains of the viruses mentioned earlier to immunize the patient against MMR infections [35]. The first dose of the vaccine needs to be given between 12 and 15 months of age, and the second dose between 4 and 6 years of age [34]. The MMR vaccination program in the United States has proven to be successful in bringing down measles, mumps, and rubella [33]. The vaccine is contraindicated in pregnancy [35].

3.1 Clinical evidence for broad protective effects against COVID-19

It has been recapitulated by Miller [36] that ephemeral protection is provided by the MMR vaccine against heterologous viral infections [37]. A study of 11,004 Italian children was carried out to analyze the effectiveness of MMR vaccinations in terms of the need for hospitalizations for targeted and nontargeted infections. About 2,302 (20.9%) children had not been immunized with the MMR vaccine, 5,392 (49%) had received one dose of the vaccine, and 3,310 (30.1%) had received both doses. The study showed lowered hospitalizations (414 in all) for children suffering from all sorts of infectious diseases. About 262 hospitalizations among nonvaccinated and 82 and 70 hospitalizations among single-dose and double-dose recipients, respectively, were reported. Only 809 hospitalizations out of 11,004 children battling respiratory diseases were reported [38]. To benefit healthcare workers, airport staff, and foreign domestic helpers, Hong Kong instituted the MMR vaccination program in 2019 and continued it in 2020. This program brought down COVID-19-associated deaths and led to zero deaths during the 7 weeks ending on May 3, 2020. In 2019, 7.2 million out of 20.26 million people in Madagascar were immunized with the MMR vaccine, and as of May 4, 2020, no deaths were reported of patients suffering from COVID-19 [39].

It is mandatory for every man from South Korea between 18 and 28 years of age to join the South Korean military due to the country's new vaccination policy formed by the 2012 Military Healthcare Services Act. Every recruit compulsorily receives two doses of MMR vaccine apart from childhood immunizations, and maximum immunity can be witnessed among these individuals. South Korea also vaccinated its entire population post measles outbreak in 2001–2002. South Korea has shown an unusually low incidence of deaths due to COVID-19 as compared with other countries with a similar timeline of initial infection [39, 40].

A study of 2,135 pediatric patients with COVID-19 in China reveals that over 90% of the patients displayed mild or moderate symptoms or were asymptomatic [41]. As per the data dated March 18, 2020, the Korean Center for Disease Control and Prevention states that only 1.03% of the total 8,413 COVID-19 cases included children as patients. These data expound on the benefit of MMR vaccination in producing innate immunity, making children less prone to COVID-19 [42]. Immunization with the MMR vaccine successfully curbs pulmonary inflammation and sepsis, which is one of the prominent causes of COVID-19 mortality and confers protection to children from COVID-19 by making them less susceptible to this horrid disease [43].

Until April 30, 2020, 1,102 people on the U.S.S Roosevelt had tested positive for COVID-19, wherein only one death and seven hospitalizations were reported. This could be attributed to the fact that all recruits are provided MMR vaccinations by the U.S. military before their admission. The hospitalization rate for Navy recruits was about 20 times lower than that for the usual population of the same age group. Another example to substantiate the correlation between MMR vaccination and the COVID-19 death rate is the lack of sufficient MMR vaccination in Italy, which has proven controversial and inconsistent [44], leading to a vast measles outbreak in 2017 that also justifies a higher death rate due to COVID-19 [39].

Pediatric patients in China older than 1 year manifested mild symptoms, whereas those of a year or less exhibited severe symptoms [45]. Introducing a dose of MMR after a year post-birth explains the study's result in China [46].

According to Roser, up until May 14, 2020, 4,477,573 cases and 299,958 deaths worldwide due to COVID-19 were reported, while only 2.2% of the cases involved children between 0 and 17 years of age [37]. It has also been reiterated by Verdoni that the course of COVID-19 involving respiratory problems is benign [47]. These pieces of evidence lean toward the possibility of boosted immunity by MMR vaccine, offering protection against COVID-19.

In North Korea, Turkmenistan, Cook Islands, Marshall Islands, Solomon Islands, and Tuvalu, many adults between the ages 29–45 receiving MMR immunizations reported zero or near-zero deaths from COVID-19 [39].

Using epidemiological parameters such as the fraction of undocumented infections and their contagiousness previously estimated from US county-level data between February 21, 2020 and March 13, 2020, [48], an SEIR model has been put up priming large populations in the United States and China to estimate spread and growth of the virus [49, 50]. Priming has reduced the infection period and chance of complications by 33%, and after the priming agent was administered slightly before the infection rate peaked, the rate of hospitalizations reduced to 25%.

In order to prevent the immune pathology in severe COVID-19 cases, some suggest that the immune system could be primed with live attenuated viruses in vaccines such as MMR, which could trigger trained innate immunity [50].

3.2 Basis of broad protective effects against COVID-19

S-glycoprotein is an immunogenic protein encoded by SARS-CoV-2 that plays a pivotal role in binding to the ACE2 receptor on the epithelial cells of the respiratory system [51]. Since MMR immunization confers broad immunity against viral infections, it has been postulated that there might be similarities between antigenic epitopes of surface proteins of the live attenuated viruses used in the MMR vaccine and the S-glycoprotein. Thus, the antibodies produced by MMR vaccination could cross-react with antigenic epitopes of the S-glycoprotein and could also provide cross-protection against COVID-19 [42].

A homology search was carried out for the chain A amino acid sequence of SAR-COV-2 S-glycoprotein against the proteomic sequences of live attenuated viruses in MMR vaccines. Fusion (F1) glycoprotein of the measles virus and E-glycoprotein of the rubella virus shared similarities in 30 amino acid residues with the S-glycoprotein. More experimental data are required in this area [42].

Lymphopenia and a decrease in cytotoxic CD8+ T cells are exhibited in patients suffering from COVID-19 [52]. Upon routine childhood immunization, secretion of many cytokines such as IL-2, IL-12, and IFN gets induced post CD4+ T helper 1 cell stimulation, which then provokes maturation of CD8+ T cells. This also elevates cytotoxicity of NK cells, destroying cells infected with coronavirus [45].

Pattern recognition receptors (PPRS) recognize viral components such as viral nucleic acids and proteins, eliciting innate immune response [53, 54]. A response to the respiratory infection due to coronavirus has been elicited by endosomal toll-like receptors 3, 7, and 8 and intracellular cytosolic PRRS. The above key sensors trigger a downstream signaling cascade, leading to the induction of IFN secretion, which activates thousands of IFN-stimulated genes, generating an antiviral response and eventually protecting the patient from harm immunopathology [50].

3.3 The current status

The benefits of the MMR vaccine, coupled with its FDA approval, ease of administration, cost-effectiveness, and availability, indicate an advantage to vaccinating the population to spare mortality associated with COVID-19 to a certain extent [55].

A randomized clinical trial with MMR vaccine for healthcare workers and first responders has been proposed to be performed in New Orleans to corroborate the data [43].

The MMR vaccination triggers innate immunity by inducing IFN secretion and escalating cytotoxicity of NK cells [45]. However, treatment with therapeutic interferons is costly. It leads to undesirable side effects, while vaccine-induced IFNS and NK cells are more robust, efficient, and potent, suggesting the use of MMR vaccination, which confers antibody-mediated cross-protection for prevention or amelioration of SARS-CoV-2 infection [55, 56].

The SARS-CoV-2 virus has an incubation period of approximately 5 days and up to 14 days and longer [57, 58] and is thought to evade the innate immune system causing delay or suppression of antiviral responses [50]. Priming the individual with MMR vaccine before the infection would trigger a broad innate immune response, which would prevent immune system evasion by the virus and prepare a susceptible individual to counter the viral attack [50].

Even though COVID-19 is affecting individuals of all age groups, it is evident that children, who are being less commonly affected by the disease and show mild symptoms, are associated with a low COVID-19-death rate and can recover faster compared with other age groups owing to the routine MMR vaccination that boosts immunity and confers cross-protection [59]. Commonalities shared by MMR viruses and SARS-CoV-2 in terms of primary replication in the upper respiratory tract [55], structural and functional similarities between them, cross-protection offered by MMR vaccine, and age-related declining immunogenicity of measles vaccine suggest the use of MMR vaccine for prophylaxis or to avoid severe complications in COVID-19-positive individuals and eventually limit COVID-19 death rates [60].

Countries such as Australia and Belgium lack mandatory vaccination programs [61]. The vaccine offers protection against measles, mumps, and rubella for 10–12 years [59]. The first dose is administered between 12 and 15 months of age, while the second dose is administered between 4 and 6 years of age [34].

Currently, WHO has not yet recommended putting MMR vaccination in use for the ongoing pandemic because of the lack of concrete evidence about the cause-and-effect relationship between the MMR vaccine and SARS-CoV-2. Sufficient evidence of the efficacy of the vaccine against this disease will pave the way to begin the mass production of the vaccine to fight the pandemic.

4. Opinion on repurposing BCG vaccine and MMR vaccine for COVID-19

There is a tremendous spike in the number of cases of COVID-19 across the globe, which calls for an emergency and fruitful strategy that would cause a flattening of the curve while saving the lives of vulnerable populations or people with comorbidities who are more susceptible to this disease. While there is a call for research aiming to develop specific vaccines, vaccine repositioning has not taken a backseat. With vaccines such as BCG and MMR showing considerable evidence for their inherent ability to resist various infections, alongside their well-established safety and efficacy for their target infections, there is great promise for a new development to combat the existing pandemic [4, 5, 12, 33, 38].

The broad protective effect of both BCG and MMR vaccines has been clinically proven. Their effect lasts nearly 10 years. BCG vaccination has been impactful in reducing mortality associated with various diseases as per studies conducted across Sweden and West Africa. Its long-lasting effect was observed in a study based in Spain, whereas protection against upper respiratory infections was depicted in a study based in Indonesia involving citizens above the age of 60. Two randomized clinical trials are in progress in Holland and Australia to study BCG's effects on COVID-19. A link between COVID-19-related mortality and the BCG index has been observed, where an increase in the index has shown a decrease in mortality in European countries [16]. Most Asian countries such as Japan, China, Korea, India, and the Russian

Federation have continued to conduct childhood BCG vaccination compared with countries such as the United States, Canada, Italy, and the Netherlands. Compared with the countries with no mandatory mass BCG vaccination, the per capita death rate associated with COVID-19 in the countries mentioned above is lower [28]. Many of these countries incorporate BCG vaccines containing original strains compared with the European countries. Currently, a study in Germany is assessing the effects of a modified strain of BCG against COVID-19.

Few countries such as Australia and Belgium lack a mandatory MMR vaccination program. A study in Italy showed a reduction in the hospitalization of children associated with respiratory diseases because of MMR vaccination [38]. MMR vaccination programs for front-line workers in Hong Kong, Madagascar, the South Korean military, the U.S. military, adults of North Korea, Turkmenistan, Cook Islands, Marshall Islands, Solomon Islands, and Tuvalu have brought down COVID-19-associated deaths in such regions. Most of the vaccinated children in China were asymptomatic or showed mild/moderate symptoms of COVID-19. A randomized clinical trial with MMR vaccine for healthcare workers and first responders has been proposed in New Orleans. The MMR vaccine plays a key role in limiting pulmonary inflammation, a key factor in SARS-CoV-2 mortality [43]. It has reduced the impact of COVID-19 because of the structural similarity between glycoproteins of COVID-19 virus and measles and rubella viruses. The SARS-CoV-2 virus has an incubation period of approximately 5 days and up to 14 days. So, priming the individual with MMR vaccine before infection can trigger a broad innate immune response, preventing immune system invasion by the virus and preparing a susceptible individual to counter the viral attack.

The BCG vaccine can confer trained immunity against many viral infections. Therapeutic interferons are expensive. Both BCG and MMR vaccines trigger the production of IFN and various cytokines, lessening the need for interferon administration [55, 56].

For the time being, MMR appears to show more human data for COVID-19 protection than BCG [39, 42]. With no concrete evidence of BCG- or MMR-conferred protection against COVID-19, WHO refrains from advising the use of such vaccines to cope with it, especially to avoid unforeseen consequences that may include upregulation of the immune system contributing to exacerbation of one's condition. Also, a surge in its sudden demand may cause a shortage of its supplies and an inability to meet the needs of infants and newborns.

5. Conclusion

The BCG and MMR vaccines require randomized clinical trials before they can be considered for repositioning against COVID-19. However, past evidence of the vaccines' ability to support to confer cross-protection against multiple viral infections can become a basis for their candidature for prospective clinical trials. Overall, the vaccines may shorten the duration of infection, minimize the harmful pathology, reduce the hospitalization rates, and help flatten the curve, helping to curb the spread of the disease. More research needs to be done to assess the risks and adverse effects of this method, especially for the elderly and people with comorbidities prone to severe complications due to COVID-19. Until there is evidence stating a direct cause-and-effect relationship between COVID-19 and BCG/MMR vaccine, the world will have to wait.

Acknowledgements

Authors are very much thankful to Dr. Paraag Gide, Principal, Hyderabad (Sindh) National Collegiate Board's Dr. L. H. Hiranandani College of Pharmacy, Ulhasnagar, for his continuous support, guidance, and encouragement.

Funding

None.

Conflict of interest

The author(s) declare that there is no conflict of interest regarding publication of this article.

Availability of data and materials

The data supporting the findings of the article will be made available from the corresponding author [Dr. Harshal Ashok Pawar] upon reasonable request.

Abbreviations

COVID-19	Coronavirus disease 2019
BCG	Bacillus Calmétte Guerin
MMR	Measles, Mumps, and Rubella
SARS-CoV-2	Severe Acute Respiratory Syndrome Coronavirus 2
RNA	Ribonucleic acid
S	Spike
M	Membrane
N	Nucleotide
E	Envelope
TB	Tuberculosis
IFN- γ	Interferon- γ
CD4+	Cluster of differentiation 4
1IL-1β	Interleukin-1β
IL-2	Interleukin-2
TNF-α	Tumor necrosis factor- α
MHC	Major histocompatibility complex
APCs	Antigen-presenting cells
TCR	T-cell receptor
CD28	Cluster of differentiation 28
B7-1	Binding protein
LFA-1	Lymphocytes function associated antigen-1
ICAM-1	Intercellular adhesion molecule-1
H1N1	Swine flu
WHO	World Health Organization

U.S.	United States
GDP	Gross Domestic Product
U.S.S	United States Ship
SEIR	Susceptible-Exposed-Infectious-Recovered
ACE2	Angiotensin-converting enzyme 2
F1	Fusion
CD8+	Cluster of differentiation 8
NK	Natural Killer Cells
PPRS	Pattern Recognition Receptors
FDA	Food and Drug Administration

Author details

Kasturi Mahesh Tawde[1], Aditya Manivannan Iyer[2] and Harshal Ashok Pawar[3]*

1 Master of Science in Pharmaceutical Sciences, Campbell University, Buies Creek, NC, USA

2 Dr. L.H. Hiranandani College of Pharmacy, Maharashtra, India

3 Department of Pharmacognosy/Quality Assurance, Dr. L.H. Hiranandani College of Pharmacy, Maharashtra, India

*Address all correspondence to: harshal.pawar@dlhhcop.org

References

[1] Rajarshi K, Chatterjee A, Ray S. BCG vaccination strategy implemented to reduce the impact of COVID-19: Hype or hope? Medical Drug Discovery. 2020;7:100049

[2] Wu F, Zhao S, Yu B, Chen YM, Wang W, Song ZG, et al. A new coronavirus associated with human respiratory disease in China. Nature. 2020;**579**(7798):265-269

[3] Shang W, Yang Y, Rao Y, Rao X. The outbreak of SARS-CoV-2 pneumonia calls for viral vaccines. NPJ Vaccines. 2020;**5**(1):18

[4] Abdallah AM, Behr MA. Evolution and strain variation in BCG. In: Gagneux S, editor. Strain Variation in the *Mycobacterium tuberculosis* Complex: Its Role in Biology, Epidemiology and Control. Advances in Experimental Medicine and Biology. Vol. 1019. Cham.: Springer; 2017. pp. 155-169

[5] Dye C. Making wider use of the world's most widely used vaccine: Bacille Calmette-Guerin revaccination reconsidered. Journal of Royal Society of Interface. 2013;**10**(87):20130365

[6] Fine PE. BCG vaccination against tuberculosis and leprosy. British Medical Bulletin. 1988;**44**(3):691-703

[7] Colditz GA, Berkey CS, Mosteller F, Brewer TF, Wilson ME, Burdick E, et al. The efficacy of bacillus Calmette-Guerin vaccination of newborns and infants in the prevention of tuberculosis: Meta-analyses of the published literature. Pediatrics. 1995;**96**(1 Pt 1):29-35

[8] Udani PM. BCG vaccination in India and tuberculosis in children: Newer facets. Indian Journal of Pediatrics. 1994;**61**(5):451-462

[9] Mangtani P, Abubakar I, Ariti C, Beynon R, Pimpin L, Fine PE, et al. Protection by BCG vaccine against tuberculosis: A systematic review of randomized controlled trials. Clinical Infectious Diseases. 2014;**58**(4):470-480

[10] Näslund C. Resultats des experiences de vaccination par le BCG poursuivies dans le Norrbotten (Suède) (Septembre 1927–Décembre 1931). Paris: Institut Pasteur; 1932. pp. 274-281

[11] Garly ML, Martins CL, Balé C, Baldé MA, Hedegaard KL, Gustafson P, et al. BCG scar and positive tuberculin reaction associated with reduced child mortality in West Africa. A non-specific beneficial effect of BCG? Vaccine. 2003;**21**(21-22):2782-2790

[12] de Castro MJ, Pardo-Seco J, Martinón-Torres F. Nonspecific (heterologous) protection of neonatal BCG vaccination against hospitalization due to respiratory infection and sepsis. Clinical Infectious Diseases. 2015;**60**(11):1611-1619

[13] US National Library of Medicine. Reducing health care workers absenteeism in covid-19 pandemic through BCG vaccine (BCG-CORONA), ClinicalTrials.gov. 2020. Available from: https://clinicaltrials.gov/ct2/show/NCT04328441. [Accessed: April 15 2020]

[14] US National Library of Medicine. BCG vaccination to protect healthcare workers against COVID-19 (BRACE), ClinicalTrials.gov 2020. Available from: https://clinicaltrials.gov/ct2/show/NCT04327206. [Accessed: April 15, 2020]

[15] Datau EA, Sultana A, Mandang VV, Jim E. The efficacy of Bacillus

Calmette-Guerin vaccinations for the prevention of acute upper respiratory tract infection in the elderly. Acta Medica Indonesia. 2011;**43**(3):185-190

[16] Escobar LE, Molina-Cruz A, Barillas-Mury C. BCG vaccine protection from severe coronavirus disease 2019 (COVID-19). Proceedings of the National Academy of Sciences of the United States of America. 2020;**117**(30):17720-17726

[17] Aaby P, Roth A, Ravn H, Napirna BM, Rodrigues A, Lisse IM, et al. Randomized trial of BCG vaccination at birth to low-birth-weight children: Beneficial non-specific effects in the neonatal period? The Journal of Infectious Diseases. 2011;**204**(2):245-252

[18] Mathurin KS, Martens GW, Kornfeld H, Welsh RM. CD4 T-cell-mediated heterologous immunity between mycobacteria and poxviruses. Journal of Virology. 2009;**83**(8):3528-3539

[19] Kleinnijenhuis J, Quintin J, Preijers F, Benn CS, Joosten LA, Jacobs C, et al. Long-lasting effects of BCG vaccination on both heterologous Th1/Th17 responses and innate trained immunity. Journal of Innate Immunity. 2014;**6**(2):152-158

[20] Li L, Qiao D, Zhang X, Liu Z, Wu C. The immune responses of central and effector memory BCG-specific CD4+ T cells in BCG-vaccinated PPD+ donors were modulated by Treg cells. Immunobiology. 2011;**216**(4):477-484

[21] DesJardin LE, Kaufman TM, Potts B, Kutzbach B, Yi H, Schlesinger LS. Mycobacterium tuberculosis-infected human macrophages exhibit enhanced cellular adhesion with increased expression of LFA-1 and ICAM-1 and reduced expression and/or function of complement receptors, FcgammaRII and the mannose receptor. Microbiology (Reading). 2002;**148**(Pt 10):3161-3171

[22] Spencer JC, Ganguly R, Waldman RH. Nonspecific protection of mice against influenza virus infection by local or systemic immunization with Bacille Calmette-Guérin. The Journal of Infectious Diseases. 1977;**136**(2):171-175

[23] Ratzan KR, Musher DM, Keusch GT, Weinstein L. Correlation of increased metabolic activity, resistance to infection, enhanced phagocytosis, and inhibition of bacterial growth by macrophages from listeria- and BCG-infected mice. Infection and Immunity. 1972;**5**(4):499-504

[24] Leentjens J, Kox M, Stokman R, Gerretsen J, Diavatopoulos DA, van Crevel R, et al. BCG vaccination enhances the immunogenicity of subsequent influenza vaccination in healthy volunteers: A randomized, placebo-controlled pilot study. The Journal of Infectious Diseases. 2015;**212**(12):1930-1938

[25] Bacille Calmette-Guérin (BCG) vaccination and COVID-19 [Internet]. Who.int. 2020. Available from: https://www.who.int/news-room/commentaries/detail/bacille-calmette-gu%C3%A9rin-(bcg)-vaccination-and-covid-19. [Accessed: August 18, 2020]

[26] Curtis N, Sparrow A, Ghebreyesus TA, Netea MG. Considering BCG vaccination to reduce the impact of COVID-19. Lancet. 2020;**395**(10236):1545-1546

[27] Pollard AJ, Finn A, Curtis N. Non-specific effects of vaccines: Plausible and potentially important, but implications uncertain. Archives of Disease in Childhood. 2017;**102**(11):1077-1081

[28] Iwasaki A, Grubaugh ND. Why does Japan have so few cases of

COVID-19? EMBO Molecular Medicine. 2020;**12**(5):e12481

[29] Redelman-Sidi G. Could BCG be used to protect against COVID-19? Nature Reviews. Urology. 2020;**17**(6):316-317

[30] de Vrieze J. Can a century-old TB vaccine steel the immune system against the new coronavirus? Science. 2020;**369**:6507

[31] Shet A, Ray D, Malavige G, Santosham M, Bar-Zeev N. Differential COVID-19-attributable mortality and BCG vaccine use in countries. medRxiv. 2020

[32] Alice Zwerling M. BCG world atlas. Bcgatlas.org. http://www.bcgatlas.org/index.php. 2020. [Accessed: August 18, 2020]

[33] Geier DA, Geier MR. Pediatric MMR vaccination safety. International Pediatrics. 2003;**18**(2):203-208

[34] Bowes J. Measles, misinformation, and risk: Personal belief exemptions and the MMR vaccine. Journal of Law and the Biosciences. 2016;**3**(3):718-725

[35] Observed rate of vaccine reactions measles, mumps and rubella vaccines, Information Sheet. 2014. Available from: https://www.who.int/vaccine_safety/initiative/tools/MMR_vaccine_rates_information_sheet.pdf?ua=1

[36] Miller E, Andrews N, Waight P, Taylor B. Bacterial infections, immune overload, and MMR vaccine. Measles, mumps, and rubella. Archives of Disease in Childhood. 2003;**88**(3):222-223

[37] Dowling C. Does the measles, mumps and rubella (MMR) vaccine enhance one or more specific functions in children and can it help against this novel paediatric inflammatory multisystem syndrome? Journal of Biological Science & Research. 2020;**2**:2

[38] La Torre G, Saulle R, Unim B, Meggiolaro A, Barbato A, Mannocci A, et al. The effectiveness of measles-mumps-rubella (MMR) vaccination in the prevention of pediatric hospitalizations for targeted and untargeted infections: A retrospective cohort study. Human Vaccines & Immunotherapeutics. 2017;**13**(8):1879-1883

[39] Gold JE. MMR Vaccine Appears to Confer Strong Protection from COVID-19: Few Deaths from SARS-CoV-2 in Highly Vaccinated Populations. Berlin, Germany: Researchgate; 2020

[40] Heo JY, Choe KW, Yoon CG, Jeong HW, Kim WJ, Cheong HJ. Vaccination policy in Korean armed forces: Current status and future challenge. Journal of Korean Medical Science. 2015;**30**(4):353-359

[41] Dong Y, Mo X, Hu Y, Qi X, Jiang F, Jiang Z, et al. Epidemiology of COVID-19 among children in China. Pediatrics. 2020;**145**(6):e20200702

[42] Sidiq KR, Sabir DK, Ali SM, Kodzius R. Does early childhood vaccination protect against COVID-19? Frontiers in Molecular Biosciences. 2020;**7**:120

[43] Fidel PL Jr, Noverr MC. Could an unrelated live attenuated vaccine serve as a preventive measure to dampen septic inflammation associated with COVID-19 infection? mBio. 2020;**11**(3):e00907

[44] Crenna S, Osculati A, Visona SD. Vaccination policy in Italy: An update. Journal of Public Health Research. 2018;**7**(3):1523

[45] Salman S, Salem M. The mystery behind childhood sparing by COVID-19. IJCBR. 2020;**4**(Special Issue):11-13

[46] Steinglass R. Routine immunization: An essential but wobbly platform. Global Health Science and Practise. 2013;**1**(3):295-301

[47] Verdoni L, Mazza A, Gervasoni A, Martelli L, Ruggeri M, Ciuffreda M, et al. An outbreak of severe Kawasaki-like disease at the Italian epicentre of the SARS-CoV-2 epidemic: An observational cohort study. Lancet. 2020;**395**(10239):1771-1778

[48] Pei S, Shaman J. Initial simulation of SARS-CoV2 spread and intervention effects in the continental US. medRxiv. 2020

[49] Li R, Pei S, Chen B, Song Y, Zhang T, Yang W, et al. Substantial undocumented infection facilitates the rapid dissemination of novel coronavirus (SARS-CoV-2). Science. 2020;**368**(6490): 489-493

[50] Kolodny O, Berger M, Feldman MW, Ram Y. A new perspective for mitigation of SARS-CoV-2 infection: Priming the innate immune system for viral attack. Open Biology. 2020;**10**:200138

[51] Wrapp D, Wang N, Corbett KS, Goldsmith JA, Hsieh CL, Abiona O, et al. Cryo-EM structure of the 2019-nCoV spike in the prefusion conformation. Science. 2020;**367**(6483):1260-1263

[52] Bermejo-Martin JF, Almansa R, Menéndez R, Mendez R, Kelvin DJ, Torres A. Lymphopenic community acquired pneumonia as signature of severe COVID-19 infection. The Journal of Infection. 2020;**80**(5):e23-e24

[53] Thompson AJ, Locarnini SA. Toll-like receptors, RIG-I-like RNA helicases and the antiviral innate immune response. Immunology and Cell Biology. 2007;**85**(6):435-445

[54] Kawai T, Akira S. Innate immune recognition of viral infection. Nature Immunology. 2006;7(2):131-137

[55] Anbarasu A, Ramaiah S, Livingstone P. Vaccine repurposing approach for preventing COVID 19: Can MMR vaccines reduce morbidity and mortality? Human Vaccines & Immunotherapeutics. 2020;**16**(9):2217-2218

[56] Sleijfer S, Bannink M, Van Gool AR, Kruit WH, Stoter G. Side effects of interferon-alpha therapy. Pharmacy World & Science. 2005;**27**(6):423-431

[57] Bar-On YM, Flamholz A, Phillips R, Milo R. SARS-CoV-2 (COVID-19) by the numbers. eLife. 2020;**9**:e57309

[58] Lauer SA, Grantz KH, Bi Q, Jones FK, Zheng Q, Meredith HR, et al. The incubation period of Coronavirus disease 2019 (COVID-19) from publicly reported confirmed cases: Estimation and application. Annals of Internal Medicine. 2020;**172**(9):577-582

[59] Salman S, Salem ML. Routine childhood immunization may protect against COVID-19. Medical Hypotheses. 2020;**140**:109689

[60] Hanker VS. Measles immunization: Worth considering containment strategy for SARS-CoV-2 global outbreak. Indian Pediatrics. 2020;**57**(4):380

[61] Walkinshaw E. Mandatory vaccinations: The international landscape. CMAJ. 2011;**183**(16):E1167-E1168

Section 4

Side Effects of COVID-19 Vaccine and Hesitancy

Chapter 9

Side Effects of the COVID-19 Vaccines

Irina Magdalena Dumitru

Abstract

Vaccination against COVID-19 was one of the most important discoveries in the fight against the pandemic and saved millions of lives. As with any vaccine, side effects have been reported, but the benefit of vaccination is much more important and should be considered. The most common side effects are mild to moderate, especially at the injection site, as well as self-limiting; non–life-threatening systemic reactions and severe reactions after vaccination are rare. In this chapter, the author will describe all types of side effects related to COVID-19 vaccines, information obtained from Web of Science, PubMed, Medline, Embase, Cochrane Library, Centre for Disease Control Prevention (CDC), cdc.gov database, and Vaccine Adverse Event Reporting System (VAERS).

Keywords: COVID-19, vaccine, protection, side effects, allergic reactions

1. Introduction

The occurrence of side effects after vaccination is a normal phenomenon; most side effects are local reactions and systemic effects are usually rare [1].

The safety of COVID-19 vaccines has been closely monitored during clinical trials, but even now, during their use, both local and systemic adverse reactions occur immediately after administration and delayed reactions [1].

Several types of COVID 19 vaccines have been used or are being used (**Table 1**):

2. Common side effects

The most common local effects after vaccination are pain, redness, and swelling at the injection site [3]. In a study conducted in the Czech Republic, on 922 health workers, local pain was reported in 89.8% of cases, after the administration of Pfizer-BioNTech COVID-19 vaccine [4]. Side effects after the second shot may be more intense than the ones experienced after the first shot [3].

Tiredness, headache, muscle aches, chills, joint pain, and fever (more common after the second dose) were also reported [5].

In his paper published in 2021, Meo et al. [6] analyzed the most recent and eloquent data on the side effects of the 2 RNA vaccines, Pfizer-BioNTech COVID-19

Vaccine	Trade-named	Type
Pfizer–BioNTech COVID-19	Comirnaty	mRNA vaccine[1]
Moderna COVID-19	Spikevax	mRNA vaccine[1]
Janssen COVID-19	Johnson & Johnson COVID-19	Viral vector vaccine[2]
Oxford–AstraZeneca COVID-19	Vaxzevria, Covishield	Viral vector vaccine[3]
Sinopharm BIBP COVID-19	BBIBP-CorV	Inactivated virus vaccine[4]
CoronaVac COVID-19	Sinovac COVID-19	Inactivated virus vaccine[4]
Gam-COVID-Vac	Sputnik V	Viral vector vaccine[5]
NVX-CoV2373	Novavax COVID-19	Protein subunit vaccine and a virus-like particle vaccine, though the producers call it a "recombinant nanoparticle vaccine"[6]
BBV152	Covaxin	Inactivated virus vaccine[4]
AD5-nCOV	Convidecia	Viral vector vaccine[7]
CIGB-66	Abdala	Subunit vaccine[8]
	EpiVacCorona	Peptide vaccine[9]
ZF2001	Zifivax	Subunit vaccine[7]
FINLAY-FR-2	Soberana 02	Conjugate vaccine[10]
CoviVac		Inactivated virus vaccine[4]
VLA2001	Valneva COVID-19 vaccine	Inactivated virus vaccine[4]
QazCovid-in	QazVac	Inactivated virus vaccine[4]
Minhai COVID-19 vaccine	KCONVAC	Inactivated virus vaccine[4]
COVIran Barekat		Inactivated virus-vaccine[4]
Chinese Academy of Medical Sciences COVID-19 vaccine IMBCAMS COVID-19 vaccine	Covidful	Inactivated virus vaccine[4]
MVC-COV1901	Medigen	Protein subunit vaccine[6]
ZyCoV-D		DNA plasmid based COVID-19 vaccine[11]
FAKHRAVAC	MIVAC	Inactivated virus vaccine[4]
COVAX-19	SpikoGen	Protein subunit vaccine[6]
Razi Cov Pars		Protein subunit vaccine[6]
Turkovac	ERUCOV-VAC	Inactivated virus vaccine[4]
Sinopharm CNBG COVID-19 vaccine		Recombinant protein subunit vaccine[6]
Corbevax		Protein subunit vaccine[6]
FINLAY-FR-1A,	Soberana Plus	Conjugate vaccine[10]
CoVLP		Virus-Like Particle vaccine[12]
Noora		Protein-based vaccine[6]

[1]*type of vaccine that uses a copy of a molecule called messenger RNA (mRNA) to produce an immune response.*

[2]adenovirus serotype 26.
[3]chimpanzee adenovirus ChAdOx1.
[4]vaccine consisting of virus particles that have been grown in culture and then killed to destroy disease-producing capacity.
[5]adenovirus serotype 26 for the first shot and serotype 5 for the second.
[6]the vaccine that contains purified parts of the pathogen that are antigenic, or necessary to elicit a protective immune response.
[7]adenovirus serotype 5.
[8]contains purified parts of the pathogen that are antigenic.
[9]subunit vaccines made from peptides.
[10]type of subunit vaccine which combines a weak antigen with a strong antigen as a carrier so that the immune system has a stronger response to the weak antigen.
[11]type of vaccine that transfects a specific antigen-coding DNA sequence into the cells of an organism as a mechanism to induce an immune response.
[12]molecules that closely resemble viruses, but are non-infectious because they contain no viral genetic material.

Table 1.
COVID-19 vaccines [2].

and Moderna, data published in the Web of Science (Clarivate Analytics), PubMed, EMBASE, World Health Organization (WHO), Food and Drug Authorities (FDA) USA, Local Ministries, Health Institutes, and Google Scholar. It was found that the most common reactions caused by administration of the first dose vaccine of Pfizer-BioNTech COVID-19 were pain, swelling, redness, fever, fatigue, headache, chills, vomiting, diarrhea, muscle pain, joint pain, lymphadenopathy, shoulder injury, right axillary lymphadenopathy, paroxysmal ventricular arrhythmia, syncope, and right leg paresthesia [7]; and pain, swelling, redness at the site of vaccine, fever, fatigue,

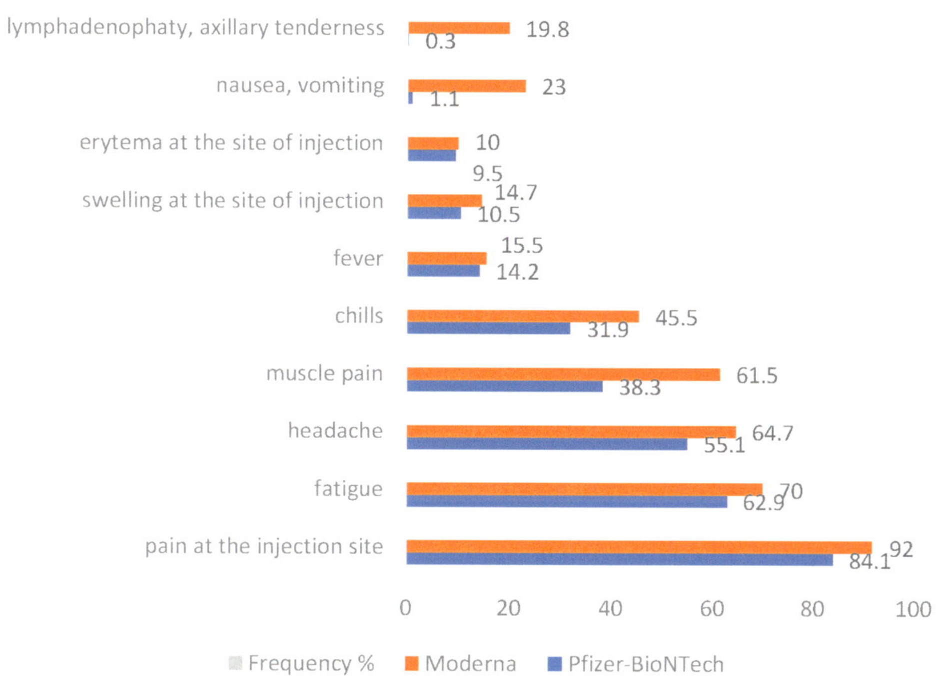

Figure 1.
Comparison between frequencies of adverse effects of Pfizer-BioNTech and Moderna vaccines [6–9].

Vaccine	Side effects prevalence	Common Side effects
Pfizer-BioNTech COVID-19	< 1 in 10 people.	Pain and swelling at the injection site, tiredness, headache, muscle aches, chills, joint pain, and fever
	< 1 in 1000 people	Temporary one-sided facial drooping and allergic reactions such as hives or swelling of the face
Moderna COVID-19	< 1 in 10 people.	Pain at the injection site, fatigue, headache, myalgia (muscle pain), and arthralgia (joint pain)
	< 1 in 1000 people	Delayed cutaneous reactions at injection site resulting in rash-like erythemas
Janssen COVID-19	< 1 in 10 people.	Pain and swelling at the injection site, redness, headache, tiredness, muscle pain, nausea, coughing, joint pain, fever, and chills
	< 1 in 100 people.	sneezing, tremor, throat pain, rash, sweating, muscle weakness, pain in the arms and legs, backache, weakness, and feeling generally unwell
	< 1 in 1000 people	hypersensitivity (allergy), and itchy rash
Oxford-AstraZeneca COVID-19	< 1 in 10 people	Vomiting, diarrhea, fever, swelling, redness at the injection site, and low levels of blood platelets
	< 1 in 100 people.	Enlarged lymph nodes, decreased appetite, dizziness, sleepiness, sweating, abdominal pain, itching, and rash
	< 1 in 1000 people	Hypersensitivity (allergy)

Table 2.
The most common reactions after administration of Pfizer-BioNTech, Moderna, Janssen, and Oxford-AstraZeneca vaccines [2].

headache, chills, vomiting, arthralgia, myalgia, and urticaria after the first dose of Moderna vaccine (**Figure 1**) [7]. Moderate or severe reactions have been reported after the second dose of vaccine, and facial swelling and Bell's palsy have also been reported [8].

Also, the most common reactions after administration of the most commonly used vaccines are shown in the **Table 2** [2].

3. Allergic reactions

Most side effects were mild and moderate, and severe allergic reactions were rare [10]. In patients who have experienced severe side effects after receiving the first dose of mRNA vaccines, dose 2 has not been given. Also, no other dose was given to patients who experienced severe allergic reactions after COVID 19 Janssen or Oxford-Astra Zeneca vaccines [10].

Documented hypersensitivity to polyethylene glycol (PEG) is a contraindication to the COVID-19 Pfizer vaccine, severe allergic reaction has been observed in about 10 cases per million doses of vaccine administered [11].

According to the Center for Disease Control (CDC), the 15-minute postvaccination monitoring recommendation is certified by the fact that most allergic reactions

(71%) occur during this period, especially in patients with a history of allergic events (81%) [11].

Anaphylaxis after COVID-19 vaccination is rare with rates of 4.7 cases/million Pfizer-BioNTech vaccine doses administered and 2.5 cases/million Moderna vaccine doses administered [12]. In cases where anaphylaxis has been reported, it has occurred within the first 15 minutes of receiving the vaccine, especially at the first dose of vaccine, usually in people who have reported allergic reactions or anaphylaxis in their medical history [13].

4. Myocarditis and pericarditis

Myocarditis and pericarditis after COVID-19 vaccination are rare. Most cases have been reported after receiving Pfizer-BioNTech or Moderna (mRNA COVID-19 vaccines), particularly in male adolescents and young adults [14]. Most of them (95%) had mild or moderate manifestations, self-limiting in most cases, and did not require hospitalization for more than four days [15, 16]. Myocarditis has been reported more often after the second dose, usually within a week of vaccination [14].

According to the Vaccine Adverse Event Reporting System (VAERS), a significant number of cases of myocarditis have been reported in young people, after the administration of mRNA vaccine, especially the second dose, with favorable evolution under specific treatment and hospitalization [17].

Related to the age group, most cases were reported in young people in the 16–17 age group (105.9 cases per one million doses) [17], followed by the 12–15 age group (70.7 cases per one million doses) and 18–24 age group (52.4 cases per million doses) [17].

In the study published in August 2021 by Diaz et al., myocarditis occurred a median of 3.5 days (IQR, 3.0–10.8 days) after mRNA vaccination, the median age was 36 years (IQR, 26–48 years), all were discharged after a median of 2 days (IQR, 2–3 days), and there were no readmissions or deaths [18].

Pericarditis developed especially after the second immunization, median onset was 20 days (IQR, 6.0–41.0 days) after the vaccination, median age was 59 years (IQR, 46–69 years median stay in hospital was 1 day (IQR, 1–2 days), no deaths were reported [18].

5. Thrombosis with thrombocytopenia syndrome (TTS)

Thrombosis with thrombocytopenia syndrome (TTS) has been associated with the administration of the Janssen COVID-19 vaccine [19]. TTS is rare and has occurred in approximately 4 cases per one million doses administered [19]. A review of reports indicates a causal relationship between the Janssen COVID-19 vaccine and TTS [20, 21].

The following features were found in relation to TTS [20, 21]:

- All side effects have been reported after the first dose of the Janssen COVID-19 vaccine (none after booster doses).

- Median time from vaccination to symptom onset: 9 days (range 0–18 days).

- 48% are women aged <50 years.
- Median age: 44.5 years (range 18–70 years).
- 83% in White non-Hispanic persons.
- 54% have a cerebral venous sinus thrombosis (CVST).

Venous thrombosis risk factors in U.S. TTS cases following Janssen COVID-19 vaccination are [20, 21]: obesity (46%), hypertension (30%), diabetes (13%), and systemic estrogen therapy (6%).

Thrombotic adverse events have also been reported following the administration of the Oxford-AstraZeneca COVID-19 vaccine, especially in younger women [19, 22]. Analysis of VigiBase reported embolic and thrombotic events after vaccination with Oxford-AstraZeneca, found a related incidence of 0.21 cases per 1 million vaccinated-days [23].

The following characteristics were found in cases with TTS in connection with Astra Zeneca COVID-19 vaccination [19]:

- TTS developed 5 to 24 days after initial vaccination.
- Women younger than 50 years of age, some of whom were receiving estrogen replacement therapy or oral contraceptives.
- Patients were known to have had previous thrombosis or a preexisting prothrombotic condition.
- A high percentage of the patients had thromboses at unusual sites (cerebral venous sinus thrombosis or thrombosis in the portal, splanchnic, or hepatic veins).
- The median platelet counts at diagnosis were approximately 20,000 to 30,000 per cubic millimeter (range, approximately 10,000 to 110,000).

6. Guillain-Barré Syndrome (GBS)

Guillain-Barré syndrome (GBS) in people who have received the Janssen COVID-19 vaccine is a very rare side effect and was reported during the 42 days following vaccination, especially in men ages 50 years and older [24].

Based on a recent analysis of data from the Vaccine Safety Datalink, the rate of GBS was 11 times higher following Janssen COVID-19 vaccination compared to Pfizer-BioNTech or Moderna (mRNA COVID-19 vaccines) [25].

In a study, conducted by Miguel García-Grimshaw and published in August 2021, on more than 3 million people who received mRNA vaccines, GBS was very rare, with incidence of 0.18/100,000 administered doses, within 30 days from first dose vaccine administration [26]. No cases were reported after second dose administration [26]. The presence of a concomitant trigger in most of our cases suggests a lack of mechanistic connection between mRNA vaccines and GBS [26].

6.1 Delayed type reactions

Delayed hypersensitivity reactions after the administration of vaccines for COVID-19 have been reported, a median of 7 days after the first vaccine dose, mainly after administration of mRNA vaccines [27]. Delayed large local reactions were noted as well urticaria, morbilliform eruptions, erythromelalgia, erythema multiforme, vasculitis, petechiae, pityriasis-rosea-like exanthems, or persistent maculopapular exanthema [28, 29]. Angioedema and liver damage were also described [28, 29].

6.2 Very rare side effects

A number of very rare side effects have been reported with various vaccines:

- A rare autoimmune neurologic disorder characterized by ascending weakness and paralysis after Janssen COVID-19 vaccination [30]
- Ocular adverse effects like facial nerve palsy, abducens nerve palsy, acute macular neuroretinopathy, central serous retinopathy, thrombosis, uveitis, multiple evanescent white dot syndrome, Vogt-Koyanagi-Harada disease reactivation, and new-onset Graves' Disease [31]
- Reactive arthritis (ReA) after CoronaVac vaccination [32]
- Auto-immune hepatitis following Covishield vaccination [33]
- Sudden sensorineural hearing loss after Oxford-AstraZeneca Covid-19 vaccination [34]
- Bullous pemphigoid rash following Moderna [35]
- Interstitial lung disease after BNT162b2 mRNA COVID-19 vaccine [36].

7. Conclusions

COVID-19 vaccines are safe and effective; most side effects are mild and moderate and resolve in a few days. Severe reactions after vaccination are rare; however, the benefit of vaccination is much greater than the risk.

Author details

Irina Magdalena Dumitru
Ovidius University of Constanta, Clinical Infectious Diseases Hospital Constanta, Romanian Academy of Romanian Scientists, Romania

*Address all correspondence to: dumitrui@hotmail.com

References

[1] Safety of COVID-19 Vaccines. Available from: https://www.cdc.gov/coronavirus/2019-ncov/vaccines/safety/adverseevents.html?msclkid=b3bdd72ecef511eca44fe7d67523108e. [Accessed: May 22, 2022]

[2] List of COVID-19 vaccine authorizations. Available from: https://en.wikipedia.org/wiki/List_of_COVID-19_vaccine_authorizations. [Accessed: May 22, 2022]

[3] Possible Side Effects After Getting a COVID-19 Vaccine. Updated January 12, 2022. Available from: https://www.cdc.gov/coronavirus/2019-ncov/vaccines/expect/after.html. [Accessed: May 22, 2022]

[4] Abanoub R, Andrea P, Sameh A, Jitka K, Michal K, Miloslav K. Prevalence of COVID-19 vaccine side effects among Healthcare Workers in the Czech Republic. Journal of Clinical Medicine. 2021;**10**(7):1428

[5] Comirnaty: Product Information. European Medicines Agency (EMA). December 24, 2020. Available from: https://www.ema.europa.eu/en/medicines/human/EPAR/comirnaty. [Accessed: May 22, 2022]

[6] Meo SA, Bukhari IA, Akram J, Meo AS, Klonoff DC. COVID-19 vaccines: Comparison of biological, pharmacological characteristics and adverse effects of Pfizer/BioNTech and Moderna Vaccines. European Review for Medical and Pharmacological Sciences. 2021;**25**(3):1663-1669

[7] Polack FP, Thomas SJ, Kitchin N, Absalon J, Gurtman A, Lockhart S, et al. C4591001 clinical trial group. safety and efficacy of the BNT162b2 mRNA Covid-19 vaccine. The New England Journal of Medicine. 2020;**383**:2603-2615

[8] Centre for Disease Control Prevention (CDC). Information about the Pfizer-BioNTech COVID-19. Vaccine. 2022. Available from: https://www.fda.gov/emergency-preparedness-and-response/coronavirus-disease-2019-covid-19/pfizerbiontech-covid-19-vaccine#additional. [Accessed: May 24, 2022]

[9] Centre for Disease Control Prevention (CDC). Information about the Moderna COVID-19. 2022. Available from: https://www.fda.gov/media/144638/download. [Accessed: May 24, 2022]

[10] Vaccines for COVID-19. 2022. Available from: https://www.cdc.gov/coronavirus/2019-ncov/vaccines/index.html. [Accessed: May 22, 2022]

[11] CDC COVID-19 Response Team. Allergic reactions including anaphylaxis after receipt of the first dose of Pfizer-BioNTech COVID-19 Vaccine - United States, December 14-23, 2020. MMWR. Morbidity and Mortality Weekly Report. 2021;**70**(2):46-51

[12] CDC. COVID-19 vaccination: Interim clinical considerations for use of mRNA COVID-19 vaccines currently authorized in the United States. 2021. Available from: https://www.cdc.gov/vaccines/covid-19/info-by-product/clinical-considerations.html. [Accessed: February 9, 2021]

[13] Shimabukuro T, Cole M, Su JR. Reports of anaphylaxis after receipt of mRNA COVID-19 vaccines in the US—December 14, 2020-January 18, 2021. Journal of the American Medical Association. 2021;**325**(11):1101-1102. DOI: 10.1001/jama.2021.1967

[14] Myocarditis and Pericarditis After mRNA COVID-19 Vaccination. 2022.

Available from: https://www.cdc.gov/coronavirus/2019-ncov/vaccines/safety/myocarditis.html. [Accessed: May 24, 2022]

[15] Heller J. Israel sees probable link between Pfizer vaccine and myocarditis cases. Reuters. 2021

[16] Kim HW, Jenista ER, Wendell DC, et al. Patients with acute myocarditis following mRNA COVID-19 vaccination. JAMA Cardiology. 2021;**6**(10):1196-1201. DOI: 10.1001/jamacardio.2021.2828

[17] Su JR, McNeil MM, Welsh KJ, et al. Myopericarditis after vaccination, vaccine adverse event reporting system (VAERS), 1990-2018. Vaccine. Jan 29, 2021;**39**(5):839-845. DOI: 10.1016/j.vaccine.2020.12.046

[18] Diaz G, Parsons GT, Sara K, Gering SK, Meier AR, Ian V, et al. Myocarditis and pericarditis after vaccination for COVID-19. Journal of the American Medical Association. 2021;**326**(12):1210-1212. DOI: 10.1001/jama.2021.13443

[19] Cines DB, Bussel JB. SARS-CoV-2 vaccine–induced immune thrombotic thrombocytopenia. The New England Journal of Medicine. 2021;**384**(23):2254-2256

[20] Shay DK, Gee J, John RSJR, Myers TR, Marquez P, Liu R, et al. Safety monitoring of the Janssen (Johnson & Johnson) COVID-19 vaccine - United States. MMWR. Morbidity and Mortality Weekly Report. 2021;**70**(18):680-684

[21] See I, Su JR, Lale A, Woo EJ, et al. US case reports of cerebral venous sinus thrombosis with thrombocytopenia after Ad26.COV2 vaccination, March 2 to April 21, 2021. JAMA. 2021;**325**(24):2448-2456. DOI: 10.1001/jama.2021.7517

[22] Lai CC, Ko WC, Chen CJ, Chen PY, Huang YC, Lee PI, et al. COVID-19 vaccines and thrombosis with thrombocytopenia syndrome. Expert Review of Vaccines. 2021;**20**(8):1027-1035

[23] Smadja DM, Yue QY, Chocron R, Sanchez O, Lillo-Le Louet A. Vaccination against COVID-19: Insight from arterial and venous thrombosis occurrence using data from VigiBase. The European Respiratory Journal. 2021;**58**(1)

[24] Janssen Letter Granting EUA Amendment. U.S. Food and Drug Administration (FDA). 2021. Reports of adverse events following use of the Janssen COVID- 19 Vaccine under emergency use authorization suggest an increased risk of Guillain-Barré syndrome during the 42 days following vaccination. Available from: https://www.fda.gov/emergency-preparedness-and-response/coronavirus-disease-2019-covid-19/janssen-covid-19-vaccine. [Accessed: May 25, 2022]

[25] Selected Adverse Events Reported after COVID-19 Vaccination. Guillain-Barré Syndrome. Available from: https://www.cdc.gov/coronavirus/2019-ncov/vaccines/safety/adverse-events.html. [Accessed: May 24, 2022]

[26] García-Grimshaw M, Michel-Chávez A, Vera-Zertuche JM, Galnares-OlaldeJA,Hernández-VanegasLE, Figueroa-Cucurachi M, et al. Guillain-Barré syndrome is infrequent among recipients of the BNT162b2 mRNA COVID-19 vaccine. Clinical Immunology. 2021;**230**:108818

[27] McMahon DE, Amerson E, Rosenbach M, et al. Cutaneous reactions reported after Moderna and Pfizer COVID-19 vaccination: A registry-based study of 414 cases. Journal of American Academy of Dermatology. 2021;**9622**:00658

[28] Ackerman M, Henry D, Finon A, et al. Persistent maculopapular rash

after the first dose of Pfizer-BioNTech COVID-19 vaccine. Journal of the European Academy of Dermatology and Venereology. 2021. DOI: 10.1111/jdv.17248

[29] Bogdano G, Bogdano I, Kazandjieva J, et al. Cutaneous adverse effects of the available COVID-19 vaccines. Clinics in Dermatology. 2021

[30] Rosenblum HG, Hadler SC, Moulia D, Shimabukuro T, John R, Su JR, et al. Use of COVID-19 vaccines after reports of adverse events among adult recipients of Janssen (Johnson &Johnson) and mRNA COVID-19 vaccines (Pfizer-BioNTech and Moderna): Update from the advisory committee on immunization practices—United States, July 2021. MMWR Morbidity and Mortality Weekly Reports. August 13, 2021;**70**(32):1094-1099. On August 10, 2021, this report was posted as an MMWR Early Release on the MMWR website (https://www.cdc.gov/mmwr)

[31] Ng XL, Betzler BK, Testi I, et al. Ocular adverse events after COVID-19 vaccination. Ocular Immunology and Inflammation. Aug 18, 2021;**29**(6): 1216-1224. DOI: 10.1080/09273948.2021.1976221. Epub 2021 Sep 24

[32] An Q-J, Qin D-A, Pei J-X. Reactive arthritis after COVID-19 vaccination. Human Vaccines & Immunotherapeutics. 2021;**17**(9):2954-2956. DOI: 10.1080/21645515.2021.1920274

[33] Rela M, Jothimani D, Vij M, Rajakumar A, Rammohan A. Auto-immune hepatitis following COVID vaccination. Journal of Autoimmunity. 2021;**123**:102688. DOI: 10.1016/j.jaut.2021.102688

[34] Jeong J, Choi HS. Sudden sensorineural hearing loss after COVID-19 vaccination. International Journal of Infectious Diseases. 2021;**113**:341-343. DOI: 10.1016/j.ijid.2021.10.025

[35] Kong J, Cuevas-Castillo F, Nassar M, Lei CM, Idrees Z, Fix WC, et al. Bullous drug eruption after second dose of mRNA-1273 (Moderna) COVID-19 vaccine: Case report. Journal of Infection and Public Health. 2021;**14**:1392-1394. DOI: 10.1016/j.jiph.2021.06.021

[36] Yoshifuji A, Ishioka K, Masuzawa Y, Suda S, Murata S, et al. COVID-19 vaccine induced interstitial lung disease. Journal of Infection and Chemotherapy. 2022;**28**(1):95-98. DOI: 10.1016/j.jiac.2021.09.010

Chapter 10

Optic Neuritis Following COVID-19 Vaccination: Real-World Ophthalmic Presentation

Madhurima Roy and Charuta Shrotriya

Abstract

After being plagued by COVID-19 for nearly 2 years, the whole world wishes for little more than the complete eradication of the disease. Our country, India commenced the much-awaited vaccination drive in Jan 2021. Ophthalmic manifestations have appeared in many forms post-COVID, amongst which neuro-ophthalmic manifestations are infrequent. This is a short series of three cases that presented with optic neuritis (ON). On further inquiry, all had received the Covishield vaccine within 5–12 days before the presentation, with no history of COVID-positive RT-PCR. All patients improved after pulse steroid therapy and are still under follow-up. Nevertheless, it's hard to determine whether post-COVD vaccine ON is a coincidence or cause. This series highlights the importance of taking the history of recent vaccination, especially in patients presenting with ON in the COVID 19 pandemic era.

Keywords: COVID-19, covishield vaccine, post vaccine optic neuritis, adverse events, ocular manifestations

1. Introduction

Optic neuritis, a predominantly clinical entity that is typically characterized by a diminution of vision, loss of color vision, and painful eye movement, is an uncommon but serious consequence following vaccination. Vaccinations contributed to the eradication of many infectious diseases like smallpox, poliomyelitis, and measles in world history. Neurological events following vaccination such as seizures, encephalopathy, or GBS [1, 2], are not unheard of, with the earliest reports dating back to the late 19th century, following the development of neuroparalytic syndrome after Pasteur's rabies immunization [3]. The rapid development and availability of vaccination, ahead of an anticipated timetable, for relief from the COVID-19 pandemic, was an unprecedented and monumental accomplishment, which, consequently left the prospect and question of long-term safety open and ambiguous. A meta-analysis of five randomized, double-blind, placebo-controlled trials of COVID-19 vaccine candidates noted that local and systemic adverse events reported were all mild to moderate and transient in nature [4]. Therefore, reporting an untoward outcome following vaccination is paramount to establishing a safety threshold for widespread public usage. From January 2021 onwards, India commenced the much-awaited vaccination drive. Ophthalmic manifestations have appeared in many forms post-COVID, amongst which neuro-ophthalmic manifestations are infrequent. This review article presents a short series of three cases from the real-world scenario that presented with optic neuritis (ON), post-vaccination. On further inquiry, all had received the Covishield vaccine within 5–12 days just before the presentation, with no history of RT-PCR positive COVID infection. An improvement was noted in all the patients after the pulsed intravenous methylprednisolone therapy, as per the ONTT (Optic Neuritis Treatment Trial) study, and the patients are currently under follow-up. Although it's hard to determine whether post-COVID vaccine ON is a coincidence or cause, this series highlights the importance of taking the history of recent vaccination, especially in patients presenting with ON in the COVID 19 pandemic era. Reporting cases of adverse reactions that manifest after the vaccination is a challenging yet imperative task to allow for the sustained development and research of vaccines, which are safe and effective for public usage.

2. Case descriptions

A 27-year-old lady presented with an acute onset decrease in vision, which was progressive in nature and associated with mild peri-ocular pain, in the left eye (LE) for 5 days. She did not give a history of diabetes or hypertension. On examination, the best-corrected visual acuity (BCVA) was found to be 20/20 in the right eye (RE) and 20/200 in the LE, along with RAPD and color desaturation (3 out of 21 plates on the Ishihara chart) in the LE. Fundoscopy of the LE revealed a diffusely swollen optic nerve head (**Figure 1a**). Visual field examination with automated perimetry (AP) showed an enlarged blind spot (**Figure 1b**). On further probing, it was revealed that 9 days before the presentation, she had received her first dose of the Covishield vaccine. MRI of the brain and orbits (T2) revealed an enhancement of the left optic nerve head just behind the disc (**Figure 1c**). VEP showed a flat wave in the LE compared to the RE (**Figure 1d**) which led to a diagnosis of optic neuritis (ON) in the LE, for which a neurologist's opinion was sought. Hematological examination showed normal limits of ESR and CRP, and antibody titer (Ab): ANA, ANCA, MOG, NMO (Aquaporin4) was negative. The patient was administered intravenous methylprednisolone pulse therapy for 3 days, followed by an oral steroid, following which, there was an improvement in BCVA to 20/40 in LE and the fundus revealed a reduction in the swelling of the optic nerve head (**Figure 1e**).

A 48-year-old Indian woman came to the hospital with gradual and painless diminution of vision in the LE, for 3 days. Examination revealed a BCVA of 20/30 in the RE and 20/80 in LE, along with RAPD. On dilated fundoscopy, a swollen optic disc with blurred margins was discovered (**Figure 2a**). An OCT was done, which revealed peri-papillary swelling of the retina (**Figure 2b**). Examination of the visual fields showed an inferior arcuate defect (**Figure 2c**) and VEP showed delayed latency and decreased amplitude in LE (**Figure 2d**). On probing, it was revealed that 5 days before presentation, she had received the second dose of the Covishield vaccine. She did not have any systemic illness or history of preceding fever. A diagnosis of ON was made in LE, with indices such as ESR, CRP, MRI brain, and orbit found to be within normal limits. A neurologist's consultation was sought and intravenous methylprednisolone pulse therapy was started. On follow-up, it was found that the BCVA had improved to 20/30 in LE and AP also showed a marked improvement (**Figure 2e**).

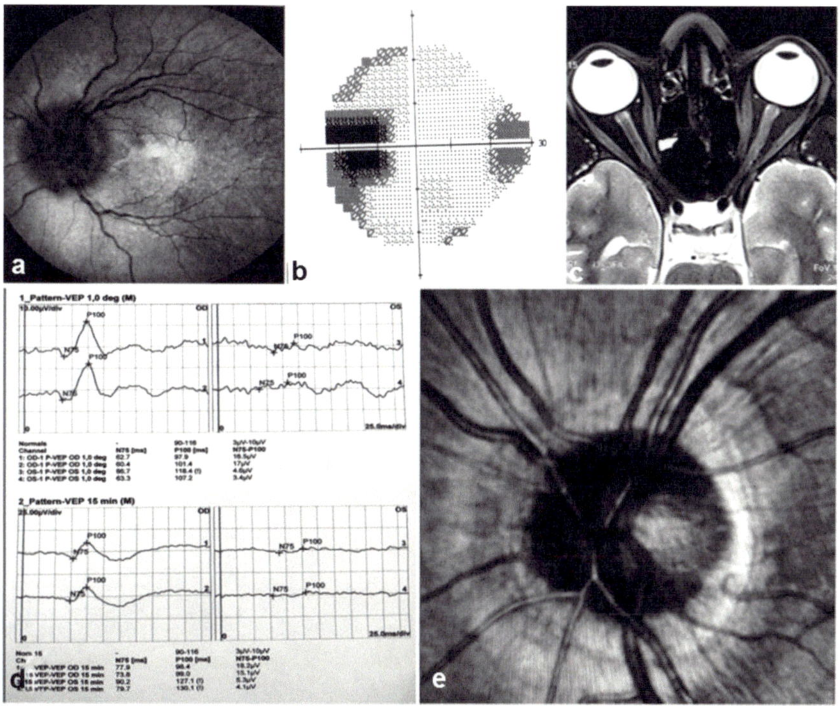

Figure 1.
(a) Fundus showing swollen optic disc with blurred margins in LE. (b) AP showing enlarged blind spot. (c) MRI brain and orbit showing enhancement of the left optic nerve. (d) VEP showing flat waves in LE. (e) Fundus picture showing reduced swelling of the disc on follow-up.

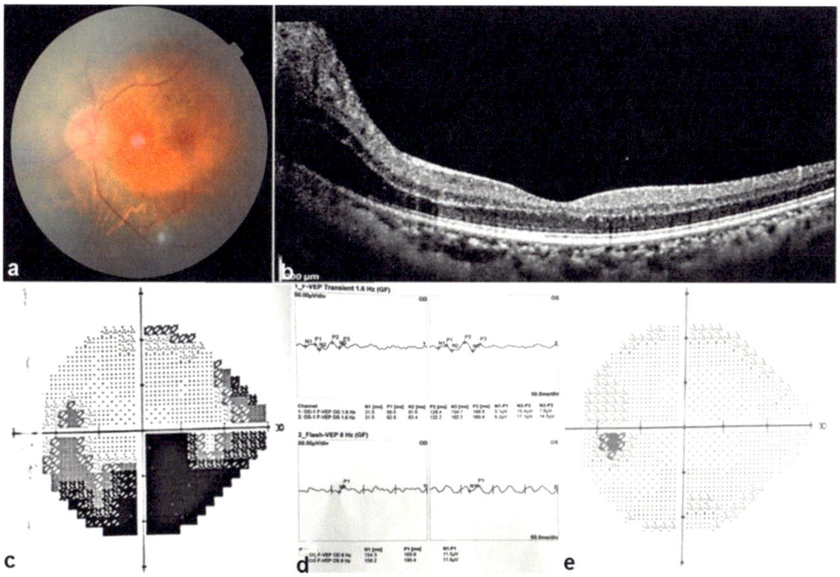

Figure 2.
(a) Fundus showing swollen optic disc with blurred margin in LE. (b) OCT showing peripapillary swelling of the retina. (c) AP revealing an arcuate defect in the inferior hemifield. (d) VEP showing delayed latency and decreased amplitude. (e) Follow-up AP showing improvement.

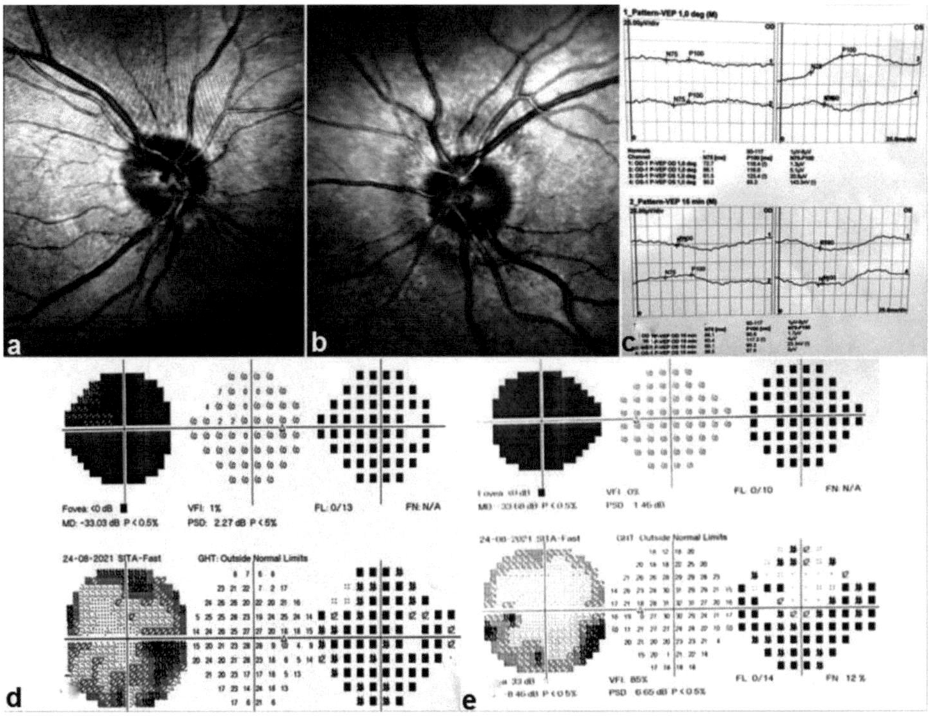

Figure 3.
(a and b) Fundus photo showing swollen optic disc with blurred margin in both eyes. (c) VEP showing bilateral flat waves. (d and e) AP showing bilateral generalized depression of field on presentation, with improvement on follow-up.

A 40-year-old Indian gentleman presented with a diminution of vision in both eyes (BE) which was acute in onset and was accompanied by peri-ocular pain for 7 days. Further inquiry revealed that 12 days before presentation, he had received the first dose of the Covishield vaccine. Ocular examination showed that the BCVA was 20/200 in BE. Anterior segment examination was unremarkable except for a sluggishly reacting pupil in both eyes (BE). On dilated fundoscopy, BE showed indistinct and swollen optic disc margins (**Figure 3a** and **b**). Visual field examination revealed generalized depression of the visual fields in BE (**Figure 3d** and **e**). VEP showed flat waves in BE (**Figure 3c**). A diagnosis of bilateral ON was made. Hematological examination revealed that ESR and CRP were within normal limits. He was started on intravenous methylprednisolone pulse therapy for 3 days followed by oral steroids in a tapering fashion after a neurologist consultation. After treatment with steroids, the visual acuity improved to 20/30 in RE and 20/40 in LE. Serial AP revealed an improvement of the fields with an inferior arcuate defect (**Figure 3d** and **e**). MRI brain and orbit was requested on follow-up.

3. Discussion

We are living amid a pandemic, where along with various systems, COVID-19 also involves the eye, including both the anterior segment, in the form of conjunctivitis, episcleritis, and the posterior segment, in the form of vascular occlusion, and maculopathy. Additionally, reports have been made of neuro-ophthalmic involvement in the form of ON, tonic pupil, and orbital involvement. COVID-19 is reported to involve nearly all systems from mild to life-threatening severe respiratory distress to even death [5]. They say necessity is the mother of all inventions, and true to the word, the COVID-19 pandemic has prompted a worldwide effort toward employing futuristic technology in the development of vaccinations at an expedited rate. COVID vaccines form a crucial step in controlling the pandemic, with over a hundred million vaccines administered since the commencement of the mass vaccination program in early December 2020. Studies and trials do not report any major safety concerns in phase 3 randomized trials [6] nor in prospective studies [7] with a reportedly minuscule number of serious neurological side effects of these novel vaccines [8, 9]. The COVID vaccine, like any other, can cause side effects including mostly low-grade fever or muscle aches, and rarely neurological events [10]. Ocular side-effects caused by vaccinations are widely studied in existing literature [11–15], and occurrence of facial nerve palsies [16], abducens nerve palsy [17], acute macular neuropathy [18–20], central serous retinopathy [21], thrombosis [22], uveitis [23, 24], multiple evanescent white dot syndrome (MEWDS) [25], Vogt-Koyanagi-Harada (VKH) reactivation [26] and Grave's disease [27] has been documented after administration of the COVID-19 vaccination. As early as 2 weeks following administration of the inactivated COVID-19 vaccination, 12 eyes of 9 patients suffered from various ocular conditions such as choroiditis, uveitis, keratitis, scleritis, acute retinal necrosis, and iridocyclitis as reported by Kunpeng et al. [28] Predominantly retinal adverse events, namely paracentral acute middle maculopathy (PAMM), acute macular neuropathy (AMN), and subretinal fluid were reported by Pichi et al., after Sinopharm COVID-19 vaccination in 7 patients [29]. In this case series, all patients presented with ON, which developed within 5–12 days (mean 8.6 days) of COVID-19 vaccination. ON following vaccination, though rare, is not unheard of. There is a certain level of ambiguity when it comes to the exact mechanism which causes ON, but an activation of the host's immune system, leading to widespread damage of the myelin sheath of the optic nerve by the host T cells, is a popularly accepted theory [30]. Any side effects after vaccination are reported to VAERS (Vaccine Adverse Event Reporting System), a passive surveillance system, by health care professionals, patients who are affected, and by the vaccine manufacturers directly. A majority of patients who suffered from ON after vaccination (229 of the reported 537 cases) were reportedly isolated events [31–33]. Predominantly reported post-vaccine ON was due to the influenza vaccine, followed by ON post HPV, HBV vaccine [34]. ON developing as early as 24 hours post MMR vaccination, had also been reported [35]. Sawalha et al. [36] reported a case of bilateral ON which occurred within a week of COVID-19 symptoms. Similarly, Zhou et al. reported another case within a few days of COVID-19 [37]. Although ON following vaccination is an uncommon side effect, safety concerns are required. Recently, following the COVID-19 mRNA vaccination, two cases of bilateral arteritic anterior ischemic optic neuropathy (AAION) and acute zonal occult outer retinopathy (AZOOR) were reported [38]. Another study reported an acute diminution of visual acuity and visual fields following the 2nd dose of Pfizer- BioNTech vaccine [39]. Following the first dose of the ChAdO_1 COVID-19 vaccine, a 40-year-old lady with a history of remitting-relapsing MS complained of blurred vision which quickly deteriorated to complete blindness, as reported by Helmchen et al., which on further investigation was diagnosed as optic neuritis with AQP4-antibody-negative neuromyelitis optica spectrum disorders-like syndrome [40].

To date, Alvarez et al. provide the largest multi-national report after vaccination against SARS-CoV-2, where 38 out of 55 cases of ON were associated with the AstraZeneca vaccine, mostly with a negative history of neuro-inflammation [41]. There was also a recent case report of the development of acute thyroiditis and bilateral ON following the CoronaVac vaccine [42]. Most of the reviewed literature includes case reports and series (**Table 1**), and there are certain limitations with regards to ophthalmic assessment, the treatment that was initiated, the visual outcome, and a general underreporting of cases.

As per the existing literature, this is very likely the first reported series of ON from India, following COVID-19 vaccination, with no evidence of an active infection. The approved Covishield vaccination was administered to all three patients, following which, two of the patients developed ON after the first dose and one after the 2nd dose. None of the patients had a previous history of RT-PCR-positive COVID-19 infection. As per the current information, Covishield is a recombinant vaccine in which, the SARS-CoV-2 spike glycoprotein is encoded by a replication-deficient chimpanzee adenoviral vector, which initiates an immunological response upon administration. A majority of the side effects occur on the day of vaccination, within 6–8 hours, but they are mostly self-limiting and resolve within 2–3 days. ON has been shown to occur due to a dysimmunological process caused by B cells targeting the adenoviral vector [45]. Although a review of safety has shown that the vaccine is generally well-tolerated, the possibility of ON should be kept in mind. A way forward can be to ask to report any new visual symptoms early, following vaccination. In our

Study	Type	Number of cases	Presentation	Duration between development of ON and vaccination	Vaccine	Age
Alvarez et al. (pre-print) [41]	Observational study, Cohort	55	27 papillitis 14- MOG +	Median – 18 days (range: 1–69)	38/55- AstraZeneca 13- Pfizer-BioNTech 4 - Sinovac	Median – 45 years (range: 18–75)
Helmchen et al. [40]		1	Optic neuritis with AQP4-antibody negative neuromyelitis optica spectrum disorders-like syndrome		ChAdO_1 COVID-19 vaccine	40 years, female, history of relapsing-remittent multiple sclerosis (MS)
Pawar et al., 2021 [43]	Case report	1	Unilateral ON	21 days	Unspecified	28 years, female
Elnahry et al., 2021 [44]	Case report	1	CNS inflammatory syndrome with neuroretinitis	16 days	BNT162b2, #2	69 years, female
	Case report	1	Unilateral ON	4 days	AZD1222,#1	32 years, female

Table 1.
Review of literature of development of Optic neuritis following COVID-19 vaccination.

series, all three patients responded well to steroids, as per the proposed ONTT trial. Although it's hard to determine whether post-COVID vaccine ON is a coincidence or cause, this series highlights the importance of taking the history of recent vaccination, especially in patients presenting with ON in the COVID-19 pandemic era.

4. Conclusion

This case series from real-world evidence, although small, can serve as a precedent for the reporting of any further cases, to secure a foothold and build a foundation for a greater understanding of whether post-COVID-19 vaccine ON is consequential or coincidental. It is prudent to ask for a thorough history of not just SARS-CoV infection but also vaccination, in a patient presenting with ON, as per the established connection. A close follow-up should be maintained to detect demyelinating disease early, in such patients.

Key summary points

1. Further, more research on pharmacovigilance and a dedicated international body for compiling any rare side effects following COVID-19 vaccination would allow for better understanding and tailored guidelines.

2. It is imperative to keep in mind, the relatively low level of side effects that have occurred compared to the vast majority of the world population who have been vaccinated.

3. Tracking of potentially harmful side effects of the vaccine can be considerably improved if ophthalmologists and physicians reported cases using VAERS.

4. The benefits of vaccination abundantly outweigh the risks and no existing literature advises against vaccination, from an ophthalmic viewpoint.

Author details

Madhurima Roy[1*] and Charuta Shrotriya[2]

1 Department of Retina and Vitreous, Susrut Eye Foundation and Research Centre, Kolkata, India

2 Department of Ophthalmology, Susrut Eye Foundation and Research Centre, Kolkata, India

*Address all correspondence to: kutunandini@yahoo.com

References

[1] Agmon-Levin N, Kivity S, Szyper-Kravitz M, Shoenfeld Y. Transverse myelitis and vaccines: A multi-analysis. Lupus. 2009;**18**:1198-1204

[2] Karussis D, Petrou P. The spectrum of post-vaccination inflammatory CNS demyelinating syndromes. Autoimmunity Reviews. 2014;**13**:215-224

[3] Miravalle A, Biller J, Schnitzler E, Bonwit A. Neurological complications following vaccinations. Neurological Research. 2010;**32**:285-292

[4] Yuan P, Ai P, Liu Y, Ai Z, Wang Y, Cao W, et al. Safety, tolerability, and immunogenicity of COVID-19 vaccines: A systematic review and meta-analysis. medRxiv. 2020;**11**:20224998. DOI: 10.1101/2020.11.03.20224998

[5] Polack FP, Thomas SJ, Kitchin N, Absalon J, Gurtman A, Lockart S, et al. Safety and efficacy of the BNT162b2 mRNA COVID-19 vaccine. NEJM. 2020;**383**(27):260315

[6] Sen M, Honavar SG, Sharma N, Sachdev MS. COVID-19, and eye: A review of ophthalmic manifestations of COVID-19. Indian Journal of Ophthalmology. 2021 Mar;**69**(3):488

[7] Voysey M, Clemens SAC, Madhi SA, et al. Safety and efficacy of the ChAdOx1 nCoV-19 vaccine (AZD1222) against SARS-CoV-2: An interim analysis of four randomized controlled trials in Brazil, South Africa, and the UK. The Lancet. 2021;**397**(10269):99-111. DOI: 10.1016/S0140-6736(20)32661-1

[8] Menni C, Klaser K, May A, Polidori L, Capdevila J, Louca P, et al. Vaccine side-effects and SARS-CoV-2 infection after vaccination in users of the COVID Symptom Study app in the UK: A prospective observational study. The Lancet Infectious Diseases. 2021 Jul 1;**21**(7):939-949. DOI: 10.1016/S1473-3099(21)00224-3

[9] Goss AL, Samudralwar RD, Das RR, Nath A. ANA investigates neurological complications of COVID-19 vaccines. Annals of Neurology. 2021;**89**(5):856-857. DOI: 10.1002/ana.26065

[10] Roman GC, Gracia F, Torres A, Palacios A, Gracia K, Harris D. Acute Transverse Myelitis (ATM): Clinical review of 43 patients with COVID-19-associated ATM and 3 post-vaccination ATM serious adverse events with the chAdOx1 nCoV-19 vaccine (AZD1222). Frontiers in Immunology. 2021;**12**:653786. DOI: 10.3389/fimmu.2021.653786

[11] Lu L, Xiong W, Mu J, Zhang Q, Zhang H, Zou L, et al. Neurological side effects of COVID-19 vaccines are rare. Acta Neurologica Scandinavica. 2021 Jul;**144**(1):111

[12] Baxter R, Lewis E, Fireman B, DeStefano F, Gee J, Klein NP. Case-centered analysis of optic neuritis after vaccines. Clinical Infectious Diseases. 2016;**63**:79-81

[13] Agarwal A, Garg D, Goyal V, Pandit AK, Srivastava AK, Srivastava MP. Optic neuritis following the antirabies vaccine. Tropical Doctor. 2020;**50**:85-86

[14] Van de Geijn EJ, Tukkie R, van Philips LA, Punt H. Bilateral optic neuritis with branch retinal artery occlusion associated with vaccination. Documenta Ophthalmologica. 1994;**86**:403-408

[15] Basilious A, Jivraj I, DeAngelis D. Acute unilateral ptosis and myositis

following the H1N1 influenza vaccine. Ophthalmic Plastic & Reconstructive Surgery. 2020;**36**:e16-e17

[16] Repajic M, Lai XL, Xu P, Bell's LA. Palsy after the second dose of Pfizer COVID-19 vaccination in a patient with a history of recurrent Bell's palsy. Brain, Behavior, & Immunity - Health. 2021 Oct 1;**25**(5):302-303. DOI: 10.1016/j.bbih.2021.100217

[17] Reyes-Capo DP, Stevens SM, Cavuoto KM. Acute abducens nerve palsy following COVID-19 vaccination. Journal of AAPOS. Oct 1;**25**(5):302-303. DOI: 10.1016/j.jaapos.2021.05.003

[18] Book BAJ, Schmidt B, Foerster AMH. Bilateral acute macular neuroretinopathy after vaccination against SARS-CoV-2. JAMA Ophthalmology. 2021;**139**(7):e212471. DOI: 10.1001/jamaophthalmol.2021.2471

[19] Mambretti M, Huemer J, Torregrossa G, Ullrich M, Findl O, Casalino G. Acute macular neuroretinopathy following coronavirus disease 2019 vaccination. Ocular Immunology and Inflammation. 2021;**30**:1-4. DOI: 10.1080/09273948.2021.1946567.30

[20] Michel T, Stolowy N, Gascon P, et al. Acute macular neuroretinopathy after COVID-19 vaccine. Journal of Ophthalmic Inflammation and Infection. 2021

[21] Fowler N, Mendez Martinez NR, Pallares BV, Maldonado RS. Acute-onset central serous retinopathy after immunization with COVID-19 mRNA vaccine. American Journal of Ophthalmology Case Reports. 2021;**23**:101136. DOI: 10.1016/j.ajoc.2021.101136

[22] Bayas A, Menacher M, Christ M, Behrens L, Rank A, Naumann M. Bilateral superior ophthalmic vein thrombosis, ischaemic stroke, and immune thrombocytopenia after ChAdOx1 nCoV-19 vaccination. Lancet. 2021;**397**(10285):e11. DOI: 10.1016/s0140-6736(21)00872-2

[23] Goyal M, Murthy SI, Annum S. Bilateral multifocal choroiditis following COVID-19 vaccination. Ocular Immunology and Inflammation. 2021;**3**:1-5. DOI: 10.1080/09273948.2021.1957123

[24] Rabinovitch T, Ben-Arie-Weintrob Y, Hareuveni-Blum T, et al. Uveitis following the BNT162b2 mRNA vaccination against SARS-CoV-2 infection: A possible association. Retina. 2021 Dec 1;**41**(12):2462-2471. DOI: 10.1097/iae.0000000000003277

[25] Ramakrishnan MS, Patel AP, Melles R, Vora RA. Multiple evanescent white dot syndrome: Findings from a large Northern California Cohort. Ophthalmology Retina. 2021 Sep 1;**5**(9):850-854. DOI: 10.1016/j.oret.2020.11.016

[26] Papasavvas I, Herbort CP Jr. Reactivation of Vogt-Koyanagi- Harada disease under control for more than 6 years, following anti-SARS-CoV-2 vaccination. Journal of Ophthalmic Inflammation and Infection. 2021;**11**(1):21. DOI: 10.1186/s12348-021-00251-5

[27] Vera-Lastra O, Ordinola Navarro A, Cruz Domiguez MP, Medina G, Sanchez Valadez TI, Jara LJ. Two cases of graves' disease following SARS-CoV-2 vaccination: An autoimmune/inflammatory syndrome induced by adjuvants. Thyroid. 2021 Sep 1;**31**(9):1436-1439. DOI: 10.1089/thy.2021.0142

[28] Pang K, Pan L, Guo H, Wu X. Case report: Associated ocular adverse

reactions with inactivated COVID-19 vaccine in China. Frontiers in Medicine. 2022:2928

[29] Pichi F, Aljneibi S, Neri P, Hay S, Dackiw C, Ghazi NG. Association of ocular adverse events with inactivated COVID-19 vaccination in patients in Abu Dhabi. JAMA Ophthalmology. 2021 Oct 1;**139**(10):1131-1135

[30] Shams PN, Plant GT. Optic neuritis: A review. International MS Journal. 2009;**16**(3):82-89

[31] Shimabukuro TT, Nguyen M, Martin D, DeStefano F. Safety monitoring in the vaccine adverse event reporting system (VAERS). Vaccine. 2015;**26**:335

[32] Roszkiewicz J, Shoenfeld Y. Vaccines and optic neuritis: Consequence or coincidence? Immunome Research. 2021;**17:1-2.3**(36):4398-4405

[33] Roszkiewicz J, Shoenfeld Y. Vaccines and optic neuritis: Consequence or coincidence? Immunome Research. 2021;**17**:1-2

[34] Michael ND, Jaffar TN, Hussein A, Hitam WH. Simultaneous bilateral optic neuritis following human papillomavirus vaccination in a young child. Cureus. 2018 Sep 24;**10**(9)

[35] Moradian S, Ahmadieh H. Early-onset optic neuritis following measles-rubella vaccination. Journal of ophthalmic & vision research. 2008;**3**(2):118

[36] Sawalha K, Adeodokun S, Kamoga GR. COVID-19-induced acute bilateral optic neuritis. Journal of Investigative Medicine High Impact Case Reports. 2020;**8**:2324709620976018

[37] Zhou S, Jones-Lopez EC, Soneji DJ, Azevedo CJ, Patel VR. Myelin oligodendrocyte glycoprotein antibody-associated optic neuritis and myelitis in COVID-19. Journal of Neuro-Ophthalmology. 2020 Sep 1

[38] Maleki A, Look-Why S, Manhapra A, Foster CS. COVID-19 recombinant mRNA vaccines and serious ocular inflammatory side effects: Real or coincidence? Journal of Ophthalmic & Vision Research. 2021;**16**(3):490

[39] Santovito LS, Pinna G. Acute reduction of visual acuity and visual field after Pfizer-BioNTech COVID-19 vaccine 2nd dose: A case report. Inflammation Research. 2021;**4**:1-3

[40] Helmchen C, Buttler GM, Markewitz R, Hummel K, Wiendl H, Boppel T. Acute bilateral optic/chiasm neuritis with longitudinally extensive transverse myelitis in longstanding stable multiple sclerosis following vector-based vaccination against the SARS-CoV-2. Journal of Neurology. 2021;**15**:1-6

[41] Alvarez LM, Ning Neo Y, Davagnanam I, Ashenhurst M, Acheson J, Abdel-Hay A, Alshowaeir D, Bakheet M, Balaguer O, Batra R, Braithwaite T. Post Vaccination Optic Neuritis: Observations From the SARS-CoV-2 Pandemic.

[42] Leber HM, Sant'Ana L, Konichi da Silva NR, Raio MC, Mazzeo TJ, Endo CM, et al. Acute thyroiditis and bilateral optic neuritis following SARS-CoV-2 vaccination with coronavac: A case report. Ocular Immunology and Inflammation. 2021;**16**:1-7

[43] Pawar N, Maheshwari D, Ravindran M, Padmavathy S. Ophthalmic complications of COVID-19 vaccination. Indian Journal of Ophthalmology. 2021 Oct;**69**(10):2900

[44] Elnahry AG, Asal ZB, Shaikh N, Dennett K, Abd Elmohsen MN,

Elnahry GA, et al. Optic neuropathy after COVID-19 vaccination: A report of two cases. The International Journal of Neuroscience. 2021:1-7

[45] Ng XL, Betzler BK, Testi I, Ho SL, Tien M, Ngo WK, et al. Ocular Adverse events After COVID-19 Vaccination. Ocular Immunology and Inflammation. 2021 Aug 18;**29**(6):1216-1224

Chapter 11

Hesitancy for COVID-19 Vaccines and Its Implications for Routine Immunisation

Mohan Kumar and V.L. Surya

Abstract

Vaccine hesitancy is a continuum, conditional on confidence (on vaccine or healthcare authorities), complacency, structural or psychological constraints, calculation or evaluation, vaccination convenience, and aspects pertaining to collective responsibility. The present chapter documents hesitancy to COVID-19 vaccination; and elaborates on factors that contribute to both hesitancy (barriers and concerns) and acceptance (enablers) rates, disaggregated by populations. We also discuss the multimodal nature of the COVID-19 pandemic and its vaccine hesitancy-related implications on routine immunisation. The pandemic and related movement restrictions or other mitigation measures, partial or complete suspension of vaccination clinics or fear of COVID-19, stress, anxiety, and depression may have limited parents' access to avail routine immunisation vaccines for their children. Also, the impact of COVID-19 vaccine hesitancy is not limited to pandemic vaccines but may continue to extend to routinely recommended vaccines.

Keywords: COVID-19, vaccine hesitancy, routine immunisation, vaccine confidence

1. Introduction

Immunisation, a key primary healthcare component and an indisputable human right, is a public health achievement of the 20th century saving millions of lives every year. Vaccines and immunisation programmes currently prevent 3.5 to 5 million deaths every year from diseases like diphtheria, tetanus, pertussis, influenza, and measles. Also, they have prevented major epidemics of life-threatening diseases since the beginning of their widespread use in the 1900s underpinning global health security. Vaccines are now available to prevent more than 20 life-threatening diseases and are a vital tool in the battle against antimicrobial resistance.

The history of public concerns about and questioning vaccines, however, is as old as vaccines themselves. Modern communication systems have only accelerated anxieties about vaccine safety and its regulation. This has resulted in pockets of people who are reluctant or refuse recommended vaccination(s), or who chose to delay some vaccines. The SAGE Working Group on Vaccine Hesitancy documented that any delay in acceptance or refusal of vaccination despite the availability of vaccination services is vaccine hesitancy. It is complex and context-specific, varying across time, place, and vaccines. Interestingly, the Working Group retained the term 'vaccine' rather than 'vaccination' hesitancy, although the latter more correctly implies the broader range of immunisation concerns [1].

It is important to monitor the reasons why a substantial number of people hesitate to receive recommended vaccinations. This allows identification of important trends over time and designing and evaluation strategies to address vaccine hesitancy and thereby increase vaccine uptake. Empirical and theoretical frameworks that assess vaccine hesitancy focus primarily on confidence in vaccines and the system that delivers them. It is essential to acknowledge that confidence covers trust in vaccines including concerns about vaccine safety, trust in healthcare workers delivering the vaccine, and in those making the decisions to approve of vaccines for a population. Vaccination behaviour can be explained by complacency (not perceiving diseases as high risk), constraints (structural and psychological barriers), the calculation (engagement in extensive information searching), and aspects pertaining to collective responsibility (willingness to protect others). These are the five main personal determinants for vaccine hesitancy [2]. To add to it would be vaccination convenience. The physical availability of vaccines, geographical accessibility, affordability and willingness-to-pay, ability to understand or comprehend that is, language and health literacy and ability of the immunisation services to appeal may affect vaccine uptake. In addition, the actual or perceived quality of the service and the degree to which vaccination services are delivered at a time and place within a cultural context that is convenient and comfortable may also affect the decision to be vaccinated and could lead to vaccine hesitancy.

Vaccine hesitancy is a continuum with those who accept all with no doubts and refuse all vaccines with no doubts as extremes (**Figure 1**). This may include a proportion who accept or completely refuse vaccines but are unsure. Between the extremes are those vaccine-hesitant individuals who accept some, delay or refuse some vaccines. While high levels of hesitancy lead to low vaccine demand, low levels of hesitancy do not necessarily mean high vaccine demand [3].

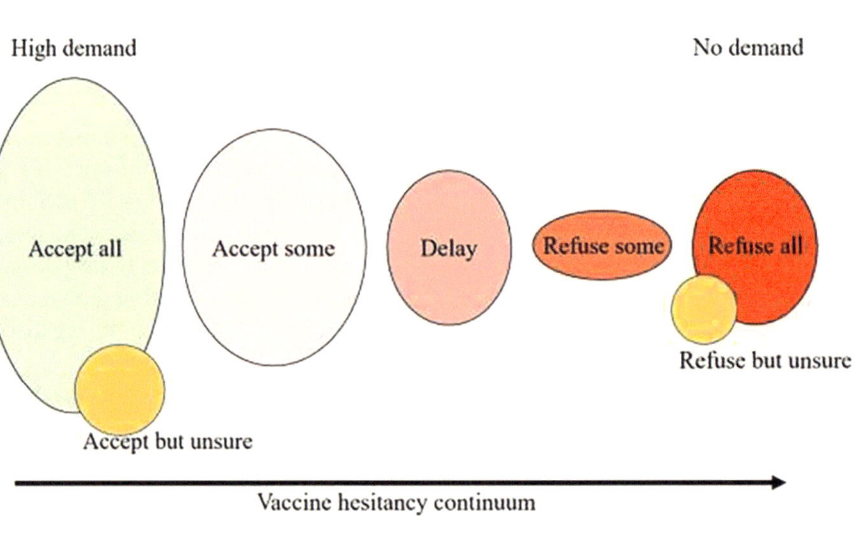

Figure 1.
Vaccine hesitancy continuum.

2. Determinants of vaccine hesitancy

Provided that vaccine hesitancy is complex and context-specific it may be influenced by historic, socio-cultural, psychosocial, family, environmental, health system or institutional, economic, or political factors. Apart from these contextual factors, individual or group and vaccine or vaccination-specific concerns may also determine vaccine hesitancy. Taking about individual and group influences, they may arise from personal or social or peer perceptions of the vaccine (**Table 1**) [3].

3. COVID-19 vaccine hesitancy

COVID-19 vaccine hesitancy is real. In a meta-analysis that computed the overall COVID-19 vaccine acceptance rate across the US, the vaccine acceptance was as low as 12% and higher up to 91% [4]. Similarly, in a community-based sample of the American adult population, it was found that the likelihood of getting a COVID-19 immunisation was 52% very likely and 22% not likely or not, with individuals having lower education, income, or perceived threat of getting infected being more likely to report that they were not likely to not going to get COVID-19 vaccine (that is, vaccine hesitancy) [5]. A multi-country study of six Southeast Asian countries showed that the majority (84%) would accept COVID-19 vaccines. However, the variation between countries was significant with the lowest rates reported in Vietnam (27%) and the highest rates reported in Russia (72%) [6]. The disparities in inter-regional and inter-country (even within countries) COVID-19 vaccine hesitancy has been well documented. In a global cross-sectional study that included participants from seventeen countries across regions, it was found that participants from China (95.3%), Australia (96.4%), and Norway (95.3%) were most likely to get COVID-19 vaccination. However, participants from United States (29.4%), Japan (34.6%), and Iran (27.9%) were least likely to get vaccinated or in other words likely to be vaccine hesitant [7]. In a nationwide survey reported from India, only 30% of adults had no issue with the COVID-19 vaccine or vaccination [8]. This finding corroborates with the neighbouring nation Bangladesh where the reported prevalence of vaccine hesitancy was 46.2% [9]. The overall prevalence of COVID-19 vaccine hesitancy among Chinese adults was modest at 8.4% (95% CI, 8.09 to 8.72) for primary vaccination and 8.4% (95% CI, 8.07 to 8.70) for booster vaccination [10]. COVID-19 vaccine hesitancy has been particularly higher among older people (27.0%, 95% CI 15.1 to 38.9) [11].

3.1 Quantifying COVID-19 vaccine hesitancy

A literature search revealed few efforts aimed at quantifying vaccine hesitancy in the population [12, 13]. Firstly, the vaccine hesitancy index (VHI) was constructed using population characteristics aligned with factors identified by an Office for National Statistics (ONS) survey analysis; the factors included in the index were population under fifty, the proportion of Black or African or Caribbean ethnic population, children under five, population with less than degree level qualification and rental housing (social or private as a proportion of the total population) [14]. This was an improved version of the earlier published COVID-19 vulnerability index (VI) that considered income domain indicators and long-term illness [15].

Contextual factors	• Communication and media environment (including social media) • Influential leaders (local or central), immunisation programme gatekeepers and anti- or pro-vaccination lobbies • Historical influences • Religion/culture/gender/socio-economic • Socio-cultural/psychosocial • Family • Perception of the pharmaceutical industry • Politics • Health and other related policies • Geographic barriers
Individual and group factors	• Personal, family and/or community members' experience with vaccination (ranging from local pain or swelling to high grade fever, to anaphylaxis) • Knowledge and/or awareness • Beliefs and attitudes in relation to health and disease prevention • Perceived or heuristic risks and benefits • Health system and healthcare providers – trust and personal experience • Immunisation as a social norm versus not needed or harmful
Vaccine and vaccination-related factors	• Epidemiological and scientific evidence in relation to risks and benefits • Organisation structure of the vaccination programme and its mode of delivery (for example, routine programme or mass vaccination campaign) • Introduction of a new vaccine or new formulation or a new recommendation for an existing vaccine • Vaccination schedule • Mode of administration (for example, oral or intramuscular injection) • Reliability and/or source of supply of vaccine and/or vaccination equipment • The strength of the recommendation and/or knowledge base and/or attitude of healthcare professionals • Direct and indirect costs

Table 1.
Determinants of vaccine hesitancy.

3.2 Predictors of COVID-19 vaccine hesitancy

The data relating to the safety and efficacy of vaccines against COVID-19 are largely from high-income countries. In addition, the rapid pace of vaccine development has been highlighted in the literature as the primary reason for COVID-19 vaccine hesitancy. A COVID-19 vaccination acceptance and hesitancy survey including data from 15 survey samples covering 10 low- and middle-income countries (LMICs) in Asia, Africa, South America, Russia (an upper-middle-income country) and the United States reported that there was considerably higher willingness to take a COVID-19 vaccine in LMIC samples (mean 80.3%; median 78%; range 30.1%) compared with the United States (mean 64.6%) and Russia (mean 30.4%). The primary reason for acceptance was explained by interest in personal protection against COVID-19, whereas concerns in relation to side effects resulted in hesitancy [16]. It is, however, important to note that reported intentions may not always translate into vaccine uptake [17]. These findings corroborate a study conducted by Africa Centres for Disease Control and Prevention, in partnership with the London School of Hygiene and Tropical Medicine, in 15 African nations. More than three-fourths (79%) of respondents in Africa would be vaccinated against COVID-19 if it were deemed safe and effective. This may be explained based on lived experience in LMICs, where many vaccine-preventable infectious diseases are still a leading cause of morbidity and mortality, resulting in a higher perceived need for or value of vaccines [18]. However, in contrast, many people including medical professionals from high-income countries have not seen the devastating effects of these diseases in their respective countries. This is because they have successfully eliminated or eradicated numerous vaccine-preventable diseases. As a consequence resulting in altered risk calculations, complacency and limited collective responsibility about vaccination decision-making [18, 19]. In a survey among the United Kingdom (UK) adults that assessed their religious and political beliefs as well as their eagerness, willingness, and hesitance to take various global COVID-19 vaccines it was found that social media use does have an effect on perceived knowledge about vaccines as well as on vaccine hesitancy (especially Twitter!). People also express concerns over the trustworthiness of foreign vaccine production and testing protocols [20].

Evidence shows that 38%, 21%, 13%, and 11% variance in COVID-19 vaccine hesitancy can be explained by vaccine confidence, vaccine complacency, sociodemographic, and other psychological factors respectively [21]. Right-wing political affiliation, higher risk propensity, and less negative mental health effects of the COVID-19 pandemic were the principal sociodemographic and psychological determinants of COVID-19 vaccine hesitancy. Other sociodemographic determinants include younger age, women, race, and employment status. However, this particular study failed to examine the variance explained by vaccine convenience factors like availability, accessibility, affordability, willingness to pay, language, and health literacy [21]. Similarly, the willingness to vaccinate among Chinese adults was associated with gender (being women), higher levels of education, married residents, increased washing hands, never smoking, a higher score of health condition, increased wearing masks, higher level of convenient vaccination, increased social distance, disease risks outweigh vaccine risk, lower level of vaccine conspiracy beliefs, and a higher level of trust in doctor and developer [10].

In a study that assessed the intention to vaccinate for different effectiveness scenarios and side effects using the health belief model, it was found that the probability of rejecting a vaccine or indecision in relation to vaccine uptake were associated with the severity of COVID-19. This includes, but not limited to, adverse side effects and effectiveness of the vaccine; decreased fear of contagion, perceived benefits including immunity, and the protection of oneself and the social environment; available information, specialists' recommendations; action signals, such as responses from ones' family and the government; and susceptibility, including the contagion rate per 1000 population. The vaccine scenarios used in the study revealed that the individuals preferred less risky vaccines in terms of fewer side effects, rather than effectiveness [22].

In a cross-sectional study that aimed at determining the predictors of COVID-19 vaccine hesitancy among pregnant women it was found that, vaccine hesitant women are younger and further along in pregnancy. COVID-19 vaccine hesitant pregnant women also reported hesitancy for influenza and Tdap vaccines. Vaccine hesitancy was associated with lack of information to take an informed decision, personal long term side effects, short and long term side effects on the pregnancy, and harmful ingredients in the vaccine [23].

In a qualitative analysis that explored the intention to receive or not receive COVID-19 vaccine among Malaysians using an integrated framework of theory of reasoned action and health belief model, it was found that the predictors of vaccine hesitancy were age, religious beliefs, subjective norms, susceptibility, attitude, and vaccine confidence or trust [24]. In contrast to the findings of a global survey from seventeen countries which reported increasing vaccine hesitancy with increase in age [7], this study reported that the vaccine hesitancy was higher among those young, primarily driven by perceived (low) risk of COVID-19. The study also stressed the importance of social influence; an individual is more likely to get vaccinated if one or the other in his/her closest circle is either vaccinated or intend to get vaccinated [24].

A population based cross-sectional study from Germany reported predictors of COVID-19 vaccine hesitancy among adults more than or equal to 18 years of age. Regression analysis showed that the odds of willingness to get vaccinated were lower for females in comparison to males; however, participants of older age group, higher education, health literacy, and adherence to preventive measures increased the odds of willingness to get vaccinated [25].

Vaccine hesitancy or say vaccine acceptance, be in at individual level or societal level is driven by complex factors. The Royal Society of Canada Framework (an adapted version of Hasnan and Tan framework) discusses COVID-19 vaccine acceptance as shown in **Figure 2**. The four major domains of factors that influence vaccine acceptance are immunisation knowledge (highlighting the importance of vaccine related reliable information, that is, easily accessible, up-to-date, and accurate tailored for each target group), healthcare workers, people in place (in accordance with the goal of the World Health Organisation Immunisation Agenda 2030) and the health care system (highlighting the role of immunisation programmes, health legislations and policies) [26]. Each of these major domains influence each other and none of these stand alone; the intersections are highlighted in white boxes. The blue circle illustrate the broader context under which each of the major domain is influenced, which includes, but not limited to, education, control of infection, communication, and communities [27, 28].

4. Implications for routine immunisation

The implications of the COVID-19 pandemic and its vaccine hesitancy against routine immunisation is multi-modal – one, the pandemic and related movement

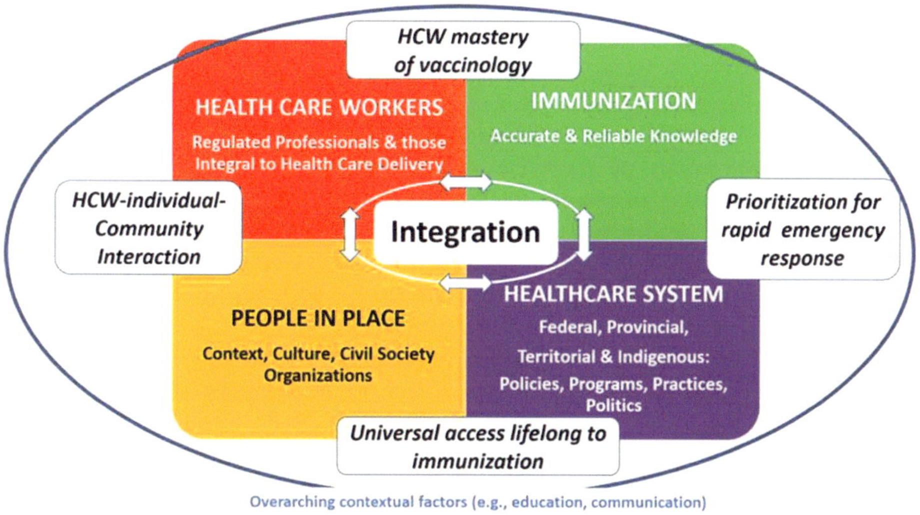

Figure 2.
Framework of factors that influence vaccine acceptance.

restrictions or other mitigation measures, partial or complete suspension of vaccination clinics or fear of COVID-19, stress, anxiety, and depression may have limited parents access to avail routine immunisation vaccines for their children [29, 30]. In a data triangulated from global, country-based, and individual-reported sources during the pandemic period, it was found that there was a decline in the number of administered doses of diphtheria pertussis tetanus-containing vaccine (DTP3) (33% fewer doses in April 2020) and the first dose of measles-containing vaccine (MCV1) (9–57% fewer doses) in the early part of 2020 [31]. The primary reason reported by WHO regional offices were substantial disruption to routine vaccination sessions, and in particular, related to interrupted vaccination demand and supply, including reduced availability of the health workforce. Similarly, a systematic review reported a decline or delay in vaccination at the time of the COVID-19 pandemic, highlighting the need for a sustained catch-up program, especially in low- and middle-income countries [32].

Secondly, the impact of COVID-19 vaccine hesitancy is not limited to pandemic vaccines but may continue to extend to routinely recommended vaccines. Though certain studies found increased vaccine confidence in parents for routine childhood vaccines as compared to the COVID-19 vaccine, certain studies highlight the concern of COVID-19 vaccine hesitancy rubbing off on routine immunisation vaccine hesitancy [33–36]. In a study that attempted to understand the impact of the pandemic on routine childhood vaccine hesitancy, it was found that the routine childhood vaccine hesitancy increased during the COVID-19 pandemic, mainly due to increased risk perception [37, 38].

It is the need of the hour to leverage COVID-19 vaccination awareness campaigns to include routine immunisation call-to-action messages [39]. Clear communication between public health authorities, providers, and the general public, and from providers to parents or caregivers on the value, safety, and necessity of routine immunisation will remain a critical piece to help alleviate concerns and address vaccine hesitancy. Engaging local leaders in the community may help resonate with public health messages related to the importance of routine vaccines, especially when the discussion around public health becomes tainted with political and/or non-medical aspects. In this process of communication, it is important to maintain a delicate balance between what is known and acknowledging the uncertainties that remain. Easing societal restrictions where possible, taking the necessary steps to reach standard marketing authorization, offering a fixed monetary reward as an incentive, involving physicians in the vaccination campaign, and focusing on vaccine effectiveness while communicating risks clearly and transparently are recommended as measures to reduce vaccine hesitancy [40].

Overall, the strategies include offering pre-structured, pre-tested communication from community trusted sources such as healthcare providers, local representatives, and authorities. It should be ensured that they are culturally relevant, accessible and in multiple languages. It is important to improve the accessibility of population to vaccines and vaccine related information. This should be made possible through adoption of flexible, context specific delivery models. The success of these strategies are rested with training and education of those involved and community engagement. It is necessary to involve youth ambassadors, healthcare workers, community champions and faith leaders to raise knowledge and awareness on vaccinations. Vaccination of friends, relatives and household members should be celebrated; an approach of community immunity should be fostered; aided by locally developed action plans with a continuous, open, and transparent dialogue [41].

5. Conclusion

The implications of contextual factors, individual and group factors, vaccine, and vaccination related factors on vaccine hesitancy is long recognised. However, the additive or multiplicative, multi-modal implications of COVID-19 vaccine hesitancy on routine immunisation is less recognised. It is the need of the hour to leverage COVID-19 vaccination awareness campaigns to include routine immunisation call-to-action messages with effective monitoring and evaluation aided by implementation research strategies. The areas that should be strengthened to restore and maintain vaccine confidence includes trust in health care provider–patient encounters, public health messaging, vaccine mandates, diversity, inclusion, and representation in health sectors, and industry influence on health care.

Author details

Mohan Kumar[1*] and V.L. Surya[2]

1 Department of Community Medicine, KMCH Institute of Health Sciences and Research, Coimbatore, Tamil Nadu, India

2 Department of Microbiology, Coimbatore Medical College and Hospital, Coimbatore, Tamil Nadu, India

*Address all correspondence to: kumar.mohan324@gmail.com

References

[1] Shen SC, Dubey V. Addressing vaccine hesitancy: Clinical guidance for primary care physicians working with parents. Canadian Family Physician. 2019;**65**(3):175-181

[2] Betsch C, Schmid P, Heinemeier D, Korn L, Holtmann C, Böhm R. Beyond confidence: Development of a measure assessing the 5C psychological antecedents of vaccination. PLoS One. 2018;**13**(12):e0208601. DOI: 10.1371/journal.pone.0208601

[3] Mac Donald NE. Vaccine hesitancy: Definition, scope and determinants. Vaccine. 2015;**33**(34):4161-4164. DOI: 10.1016/j.vaccine.2015.04.036

[4] Yasmin F et al. COVID-19 vaccine hesitancy in the United States: A systematic review. Frontiers in Public Health Systematic Review. 2021;**9**:770985. DOI: 10.3389/fpubh.2021.770985

[5] Khubchandani J, Sharma S, Price JH, Wiblishauser MJ, Sharma M, Webb FJ. COVID-19 vaccination hesitancy in the United States: A rapid national assessment. Journal of Community Health. 2021;**46**(2):270-277. DOI: 10.1007/s10900-020-00958-x

[6] Marzo RR et al. Hesitancy in COVID-19 vaccine uptake and its associated factors among the general adult population: A cross-sectional study in six southeast Asian countries. Tropical Medicine and Health. 2022;**50**(1):4. DOI: 10.1186/s41182-021-00393-1

[7] Wong LP et al. COVID-19 vaccination intention and vaccine characteristics influencing vaccination acceptance: A global survey of 17 countries. Infectious Diseases of Poverty. 2021;**10**(1):122. DOI: 10.1186/s40249-021-00900-w

[8] Chandani S et al. COVID-19 vaccination hesitancy in India: State of the nation and priorities for research. Brain Behaviour, & Immunity Health. 2021;**18**:100375-100375. DOI: 10.1016/j.bbih.2021.100375

[9] Hossain MB et al. COVID-19 vaccine hesitancy among the adult population in Bangladesh: A nationwide cross-sectional survey. PLoS One. 2021;**16**(12):e0260821. DOI: 10.1371/journal.pone.0260821

[10] Wu J et al. COVID-19 vaccine hesitancy among Chinese population: A large-scale national study. Frontiers in Immunology Original Research. 2021;**12**:781161. DOI: 10.3389/fimmu.2021.781161

[11] Veronese N et al. Prevalence of unwillingness and uncertainty to vaccinate against COVID-19 in older people: A systematic review and meta-analysis. Ageing Research Reviews. 2021;**72**:101489. DOI: 10.1016/j.arr.2021.101489

[12] Acharya R, Porwal A. "a vulnerability index for the management of and response to the COVID-19 epidemic in India: An ecological study," the lancet. Globalization and Health. 2020;**8**(9):e1142-e1151. DOI: 10.1016/S2214-109X(20)30300-4

[13] Macharia PM, Joseph NK, Okiro EA. A vulnerability index for COVID-19: Spatial analysis at the subnational level in Kenya. BMJ Global Health. 2020;**5**(8):e003014. DOI: 10.1136/bmjgh-2020-003014

[14] Daras K, Alexiou A, Rose TC, Buchan I, Taylor-Robinson D, Barr B. How does vulnerability to COVID-19 vary between communities in England? Developing a small area vulnerability

index (SAVI). Journal of Epidemiology and Community Health. 2021;**75**(8):729-734

[15] Welsh CE, Sinclair DR, Matthews FE. Static socio-ecological COVID-19 vulnerability index and vaccine hesitancy index for England. The Lancet Regional Health – Europe. 2022;**14**:100296. DOI: 10.1016/j.lanepe.2021.100296

[16] Solís Arce JS et al. COVID-19 vaccine acceptance and hesitancy in low- and middle-income countries. Nature Medicine. 2021;**27**(8):1385-1394. DOI: 10.1038/s41591-021-01454-y

[17] McEachan RRC, Conner M, Taylor NJ, Lawton RJ. Prospective prediction of health-related behaviours with the theory of planned behaviour: A meta-analysis. Health Psychology Review. 2011;**5**(2):97-144. DOI: 10.1080/17437199.2010.521684

[18] "COVID 19 Vaccine Perceptions: A 15 country study." Avaialble from: https://africacdc.org/download/covid-19-vaccine-perceptions-a-15-country-study/. [Accessed: June11, 2022].

[19] Machingaidze S, Wiysonge CS. Understanding COVID-19 vaccine hesitancy. Nature Medicine. 2021;**27**(8):1338-1339. DOI: 10.1038/s41591-021-01459-7

[20] Bullock J, Lane JE, Shults FL. What causes COVID-19 vaccine hesitancy? Ignorance and the lack of bliss in the United Kingdom. Humanities and Social Sciences Communications. 2022;**9**(1):87. DOI: 10.1057/s41599-022-01092-w

[21] Gerretsen P et al. Individual determinants of COVID-19 vaccine hesitancy. PLoS One. 2021;**16**(11):e025 8462-e0258462. DOI: 10.1371/journal.pone.0258462

[22] Cerda AA, García LY. Hesitation and refusal factors in Individuals' decision-making processes regarding a coronavirus disease 2019 vaccination. Frontiers in Public Health, Original Research. 2021;**9**:626852. DOI: 10.3389/fpubh.2021.626852

[23] Sutanto M, Hosek MG, Stumpff S, Ramsey PS, Boyd A, Neuhoff BK. Predictors of COVID-19 vaccine hesitancy and top concerns in pregnant women at a South Texas clinic [A128]. Obstetrics & Gynecology. 2022;**139**:37S-38S

[24] Ng JWJ, Vaithilingam S, Nair M, Hwang L-A, Musa KI. Key predictors of COVID-19 vaccine hesitancy in Malaysia: An integrated framework. PLoS One. 2022;**17**(5):e0268926. DOI: 10.1371/journal.pone.0268926

[25] Umakanthan S, Lawrence S. Predictors of COVID-19 vaccine hesitancy in Germany: A cross-sectional, population-based study. Postgraduate Medical Journal. 2022. DOI: 10.1136/postgradmedj-2021-141365. Available from: https://pmj.bmj.com/content/early/2022/02/02/postgradmedj-2021-141365

[26] Dubé E, MacDonald NE. COVID-19 vaccine hesitancy. Nature Reviews Nephrology. 2022;**18**(7):409-410. DOI: 10.1038/s41581-022-00571-2

[27] Hasnan S, Tan NC. Multi-domain narrative review of vaccine hesitancy in childhood. Vaccine. 2021;**39**, **1**(14):1910-1920. DOI: 10.1016/j.vaccine.2021.02.057

[28] MacDonald NE et al. Royal society of Canada COVID-19 report: Enhancing COVID-19 vaccine acceptance in Canada. FACETS. 2021;**6**:1184-1246. DOI: 10.1139/facets-2021-0037

[29] Mansour Z et al. Impact of COVID-19 pandemic on the utilization of routine immunization services in Lebanon. PLoS One. 2021;**16**(2):e0246951. DOI: 10.1371/journal.pone.0246951

[30] Rodríguez-Hidalgo AJ, Pantaleón Y, Dios I, Falla D. Fear of COVID-19, stress, and anxiety in university undergraduate students: A predictive model for depression. Frontiers in Psychology, Original Research. 2020;**11**:591797. DOI: 10.3389/fpsyg.2020.591797

[31] Shet A et al. Impact of the SARS-CoV-2 pandemic on routine immunisation services: Evidence of disruption and recovery from 170 countries and territories. The Lancet Global Health. 2022;**10**(2):e186-e194. DOI: 10.1016/S2214-109X(21)00512-X

[32] SeyedAlinaghi S et al. Impact of COVID-19 pandemic on routine vaccination coverage of children and adolescents: A systematic review. Health Science Reports. 2022;**5**(2):e00516. DOI: 10.1002/hsr2.516

[33] Temsah M-H et al. Parental attitudes and hesitancy about COVID-19 vs. routine childhood vaccinations: A National Survey. Frontiers in Public Health Original Research. 2021;**9**:752323. DOI: 10.3389/fpubh.2021.752323

[34] Badur S, Ota M, Öztürk S, Adegbola R, Dutta A. Vaccine confidence: The keys to restoring trust. Human Vaccines & Immunotherapeutics. 2020;**16**(5):1007-1017. DOI: 10.1080/21645515.2020.1740559

[35] Olusanya OA, Bednarczyk RA, Davis RL, Shaban-Nejad A. Addressing parental vaccine hesitancy and other barriers to childhood/adolescent vaccination uptake during the coronavirus (COVID-19) pandemic. Frontiers in Immunology. 2021;**12**:663074. DOI: 10.3389/fimmu.2021.663074

[36] Saurish SMVA, Amoghashree MR, Narayanamurthy, Gopi A. "Did this pandemic trigger a spike in mothers' hesitancy over their children's routine immunizations? -A cross sectional study." Clinical Epidemiology and Global Health. 2022;**15**:101023. DOI: 10.1016/j.cegh.2022.101023

[37] He K, Mack WJ, Neely M, Lewis L, Anand V. Parental perspectives on immunizations: Impact of the COVID-19 pandemic on childhood vaccine hesitancy. Journal of Community Health. 2022;**47**(1):39-52. DOI: 10.1007/s10900-021-01017-9

[38] Karafillakis E, Van Damme P, Hendrickx G, Larson HJ. COVID-19 in Europe: New challenges for addressing vaccine hesitancy. The Lancet. 2022;**399**(10326):699-701. DOI: 10.1016/S0140-6736(22)00150-7

[39] MOC Ota, Badur S, Romano-Mazzotti L, Friedland LR. "impact of COVID-19 pandemic on routine immunization," (in eng). Annals of Medicine. Dec 2021;**53**(1):2286-2297. DOI: 10.1080/07853890.2021.2009128

[40] Stamm TA, Partheymüller J, Mosor E, Ritschl V, Kritzinger S, Eberl J-M. Coronavirus vaccine hesitancy among unvaccinated Austrians: Assessing underlying motivations and the effectiveness of interventions based on a cross-sectional survey with two embedded conjoint experiments. The Lancet Regional Health – Europe. 2022;**17**:100389. DOI: 10.1016/j.lanepe.2022.100389

[41] Razai MS, Chaudhry UAR, Doerholt K, Bauld L, Majeed A. Covid-19 vaccination hesitancy. BMJ. 2021;**373**:n1138. DOI: 10.1136/bmj.n1138